Praise for *Develop Your Medical Intuition*

"This book encourages the reader to draw on natural intuitive abilities when working in areas of physical and extra-physical health, healing, and general well-being. The author has crafted a wide variety of readings, creative exercises and quizzes which are designed to develop and refine one's own intuitive powers. Drawing on elements such as auras, chakras, diet, body scans, energy balancing, and spirit guides, the book offers ways to holistically develop, refine and nurture our own intuitive abilities. Sherrie Dillard's personal experiences woven throughout the text add authenticity, and make this interesting book even more compelling."

—Bob Haddad, RTT, Traditional Thai Massage Instructor, Author of *Thai Healing Arts: Practice, Culture & Spirituality*

"Wherever you are on your intuitive path, you need to read this book. Sherrie Dillard demystifies medical intuition and reminds us each of our own intrinsic power to discern and communicate important physical, emotional, spiritual, and energetic information about our own health and the health of others. Thorough, well-written, inspiring, and accurate, this book is an absolute must-read. I highly recommend it."

—Tess Whitehurst, Author of *The Good Energy Book* and *Holistic Energy Magic*

D1521962

About the Author

Psychic since childhood, Sherrie Dillard has been a professional intuitive, medium, medical intuitive, and teacher for over thirty years. Among her international clientele are spiritual leaders, celebrities, and business executives. Sherrie's love of service combined with her intuitive ability have catapulted her intuitive practice around the globe. She has given over fifty thousand readings worldwide.

Sherrie has taught intuition and medium development classes at such diverse places as Duke University and Miraval Resort, and across the United States, Europe, Costa Rica, and Mexico. Her passion for the fusion of intuition, spirituality, and conscious self-growth has made her a popular speaker and teacher at retreats and conferences. She has been featured on radio and television for her innovative books and her work as a psychic detective, medical intuitive, and medium. Sherrie is the award-winning host of the weekly radio program *Intuit YOUniversity* on transformationtalkradio.com.

With a lifelong devotion and dedication to be of service, Sherrie has worked with diverse populations in unique settings. Along with her work as a professional intuitive, she has helped to house and feed people who are poor and homeless in New York City, San Jose, and San Francisco. She has built simple water systems in Indian villages and in the mountains of southern Mexico and Guatemala, and created art therapy programs in treatment centers for troubled youth in North Carolina and Georgia.

Sherrie holds a B.S. in Psychology and a M.Div. in New Thought pastoral counseling. Originally from Massachusetts, Sherrie has made Durham, North Carolina, her home for the past eighteen years and can often be found walking along the river with her dogs.

Develop *Your* Medical Intuition

Activate Your Natural Wisdom
for Optimum Health and Well-Being

S H E R R I E   D I L L A R D

Llewellyn Publications
Woodbury, Minnesota

FIRST EDITION
Sixth Printing, 2021

Book format: Bob Gaul
Cover art: iStockphoto.com/12254035/©gbh007
            iStockphoto.com/21725088/©helgy716
Cover design by Lisa Novak
Editing by Patti Frazee
Interior chakra border: iStockphoto.com/21725088/©helgy716
Interior chakra illustration: Mary Ann Zapalac

Llewellyn Publications is a registered trademark of Llewellyn Worldwide Ltd.

Library of Congress Cataloging-in-Publication Data
Dillard, Sherrie, 1958–
  Develop your medical intuition: activate your natural wisdom for
optimum health and well-being/Sherrie Dillard.—First edition.
     pages cm
  Includes bibliographical references.
  ISBN 978-0-7387-4201-4
1. Energy medicine. 2. Health. 3. Well-being. I. Title.
  RZ421.D55 2015
  615.8'52—dc23
                        2014048945

Llewellyn Publications
A Division of Llewellyn Worldwide Ltd.
2143 Wooddale Drive
Woodbury, MN 55125-2989
www.llewellyn.com

Printed in the United States of America

Other Books by Sherrie Dillard

Discover Your Psychic Type
(Llewellyn, 2008)

Love and Intuition
(Llewellyn, 2010)

You Are a Medium
(Llewellyn, 2013)

Discover Your Authentic Self
(Llewellyn, 2016)

Sacred Signs & Symbols
(Llewellyn, 2017)

You Are Psychic
(Llewellyn, 2018)

Author's Note

The examples, anecdotes, and characters in this book are drawn from my work as a medical intuitive and my life experience, real people, and events. Names and some identifying features and details have been changed, and in some instances people or situations are composites.

Disclaimer

The author, Sherrie Dillard, is a medical intuitive. She is not a physician or medical professional. The contents of this book are taken from Sherrie's intuition and many years of experience as a professional medical intuitive. This book is not meant to be a substitute for medical care. Always consult a physician or trained medical professional concerning any physical, mental, or emotional condition, problem, dysfunction, illness, or concern.

The intent of this book is to encourage the reader to use their innate intuition to fully participate in creating optimum health and well-being. It will provide you with the opportunity to activate and develop your natural intuition to further utilize and explore intuitive energy information as it pertains to health and well-being.

Contents

Section 5: More Tools for the Medical Intuitive Medicine Bag

Exercises, Meditations, and Quizzes

This book is dedicated to Angel Baby,
Emmalyn Alice Morris

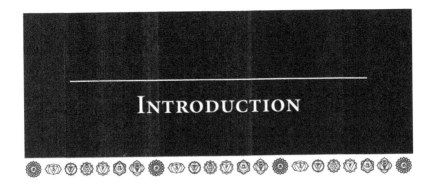

INTRODUCTION

Medical Intuition Is for Everyone

Driving into Durham, NC, from almost any direction, you will notice a sign welcoming you to the City of Medicine. As you drive into the city, it is apparent how this slogan came about. Around nearly every corner there seems to be a medical facility of some kind. I have been a professional intuitive in the area for the past twenty-five years. My office is within walking distance of Duke Medical Center and just a few blocks from the Rhine Center. Once a part of Duke University, the Rhine Center is now an independent organization that conducts research and investigates psychic abilities and other paranormal subjects. Perhaps because of this fate in location, health and wellness and my work as a professional intuitive have converged in surprising and often remarkable ways.

As a medical intuitive, every day is a magical adventure into the mystery and beauty of the mind, body, and spirit. Intuitively scanning the body for physical illness and disease and tuning into the emotional, mental, and spiritual influences that are affecting health and well-being has allowed me a glimpse into the intricate and vast cosmic network of love and wisdom that we are all part of.

Early Years as a Medical Intuitive

In my earlier years of giving intuitive readings, people asked the most basic of health questions. Inquiries into health were just one of the many subjects that clients were interested in. No one expected me to scan their body and give detailed health information. Nor did they expect that I would provide them with insight into any emotional, psychological, or spiritual issues that might be compromising their health. Instead, the anticipated responses were more along the lines of *"your energy feels low,"* or *"you are healthy."* Most of my clients were quite surprised when I told them more specific information.

In the mid-1990s interest in the possible contribution that intuitive insight could make in medical and health-related areas increased. This was in part due to the growing evidence of the importance of the mind, body, and spirit connection in healing and well-being. The role that our thoughts, emotions, attitudes, and beliefs play in our ability to heal and maintain good health was beginning to be taken more seriously by those in mainstream medicine. It was becoming more evident that nonphysical factors such as stress, negative thinking, anger, and unresolved emotional wounds lower the body's immune system and prevent healing. Mindfulness meditation, yoga, acupuncture, and energy healing were just a few of the alternative modalities that were proving beneficial in maintaining good health, decreasing pain, and healing illness.

It was during this time that a group of health professionals at Duke Medical Center became actively involved in the evolving health care landscape. In an enthusiastic gesture, Duke hosted a weekly mind, body, spirit lecture and discussion group, which was open to the public. This was the forerunner to what is now the Duke Integrative Medical Center.

This gathering of conventional and new-age types explored and discussed metaphysical, spiritual, and alternative therapies and practices. I, along with a few friends, attended as many of these meetings and lectures as possible. It was an exciting time. In the conventional and respected halls of this academic and medical environment, metaphysical, theoretical, spiritual, and philosophical experts gave lectures and shared their knowledge. Study and research groups were formed and meditation and experiential exercises were shared and practiced. One of the areas of interest being investigated was the emerging field of medical intuition. Long thought of by the scientific and medical community as mystical, unreliable, and possibly even a complete sham, intuition was receiving new consideration as a useful and beneficial tool for revealing health issues and aiding in healing.

Experiments and Further Development

Emily, a metaphysical-minded nurse, approached me one afternoon after a lecture. In the meeting, Dr. Larry Burk talked about his interest in medical intuition and the research that was currently underway. He was excited by the possibility that intuition could provide accurate information about another's physical state of health. There was lively discussion within the group and talk of future experiments.

"Let's conduct our own medical intuition experiment," Emily eagerly stated. "It'll be fun. Let's see what's possible."

Emily was enthusiastic and devoted. A client of mine for several years, I had intuitively described and informed her during our first session of the causes of a digestive problem in her son.

Emily came to my office after work on Wednesday afternoons armed with a list of patients for me to intuitively examine. These patients, whom she encountered in her work as a nurse, agreed to be part of our experiment. Although I had been giving readings for many years and providing intuitive guidance for my client's health concerns, this was a new level of professional expertise. One by one Emily recited our subjects' names and birthdays. Once I felt their energetic presence, I scanned their energy body. Patiently, Emily waited for my response. Her expectations, and my own, surpassed the depth of intuitive insight of past sessions. Emily was a serious taskmaster. She pushed me to be precise and detailed. I did not have a medical background, and I was not sure I had the ability to probe and sufficiently describe what I was intuiting. But patient after patient, we persisted.

My initial doubt was soon replaced by the realization that being able to precisely intuit the physical body in detail was easier than I had thought. My biggest obstacle seemed to be my preconceived assumption that this would be difficult. Once I relaxed and focused, I was able to systemically scan a subject's body and intuitively see and feel tumors, dysfunctions, imbalances, and illness. Problematic issues seemed to almost jump out at me. As my ability to see within the physical body increased, so did my ability to perceive and intuitively tune in to the more subtle energy body, the aura, meridians, and chakras. I began to more fully comprehend the important information contained within the multicolored and luminous radiance of energy that surrounds us.

My medical intuitive ability seemed to have a life of its own. Every day I intuitively received new health energy revelations, and my knowledge of illness, healing, and the mind, body, spirit connection increased and deepened. In the excitement of my expanding medical intuitive proficiency, I admit I became a little obsessed. I was becoming more confident, but I did not have people primarily coming to me for medical intuitive sessions. I still received general health-related questions from clients. But there was not yet a convincing general belief that intuition could provide tangible and practical help and information. At this time, I was best known as a medium, and most people came to me to communicate with their loved ones on the other side. However, my work as a medium surprisingly provided me with an unexpected but useful perspective.

It began one morning during a session. As I turned my attention to the presence of my client's mother who had passed over several years prior, I saw her energy body in specific detail. Much like the intuitive work I did with Emily's patients, my client's mother's health issues while in the physical body seemed to jump out at me. Although she no longer was experiencing any aches and pains, the emotions, thoughts, choices, and attitudes that led to her illness and eventual passing over were imprinted within her energy field. From then on I continued to begin medium sessions with the practice of intuitively tuning in to the energy body of those on the other side. This helped me to more fully realize the significance of the connection between our mind, body, and spirit and the importance of healing the nonphysical influences that lead to illness and disease.

An Expanded View of Health

After months of practice, study, and reflection, requests for medical intuitive readings began to increase. This is now a large part of the intuitive work that I do. Perhaps because of my close proximity to Duke Medical Center and the broad range of medical choices available in my town, I am not always the first medical option for many who come to see me. The medical issues of those who seek me out are often mystifying and perplexing. Under normal circumstances many of my clients would not pursue the services of a medical intuitive. Yet, for a variety of reasons, conventional medicine may not be addressing all of their needs. Some are not healing and responding to treatment. There are others who are confused after receiving different diagnoses from different physicians. A few have gone from physician to physician and are still in pain or suffering. Many are exploring alternative types of healing modalities in their search for healing. While others are simply curious. They may be acting on an inner intuitive urging or the recommendation of someone who has been helped through medical intuition.

It is through my interaction with clients such as these that the potential of medical intuition has more fully blossomed. The confusion and the persistent pain and suffering that many endure has motivated me to expand my intuitive scope. The energetic information that I regularly intuit goes beyond describing only the physical issues of health. I also intuit and share less obvious influences, such as the repressed emotions, past trauma, negative thoughts, and attitudes that may be affecting a client's health. Our relationship and career choices, spirituality and soul plan, lessons and life purpose also contribute to our overall health and well-being. This kind of energetic information is empowering. It provides my clients with a more complete picture of what influences are creating illness and disease and offers them a means to participate in the healing process. It also helps my clients to pay better attention to the intuitive health messages they regularly receive.

We Are Listening to Our Intuition

The important role that intuition can play in our health and well-being is becoming increasingly more accepted. Not only are we taking the professional advice of medical intuitives more seriously, we are also collectively listening to the intuitive health messages that our body sends us, and we are acting on this information.

This was certainly true for Teresa. An attractive woman in her forties, Teresa came into my office for her session with a no-nonsense attitude. She immediately told me that she wanted me to tell her all I could about her health. As I started to scan her body, I was immediately drawn to her thyroid and adrenals. I could feel an imbalance in her endocrine system. Her adrenals were fatigued and her thyroid looked swollen and felt dense. It felt as if she was in a kind of energetic slow motion, which was creating sleep problems, exhaustion, and weight gain. Her spirit was not in synch with her daily goals and agenda. Her soul wanted to evolve in new areas of growth and purpose. Doing everything that she could to hold on to the status quo in her everyday life, her resistance to change was physically and spiritually exhausting her.

When I described what I was intuiting, she listened, and then interrupted me.

"I know the physical state of my health," she said. "I'm a physician. I came to you to understand the emotional and spiritual issues. I know how to fix the physical concerns. But I'm not getting better. What you're saying makes sense. For several months, I've been getting the inner message that I need to take some time and re-evaluate my goals and make some changes in my life. I guess I just needed someone to verify my own intuitive feeling. I know that I've been resisting going forward."

The wise inner voice of our spirit is always communicating with us through our intuition. It is becoming increasingly common for clients to tell me that it was their intuition that led them to make an appointment with me. A health-related dream or the feeling that a loved one in spirit is sending them a message about their health compels others to take better care of themselves or to get a health checkup. More than ever people intuitively sense that dissatisfaction or unhappiness in their jobs or relationships and other stresses are at the root of their headaches, digestive problems, or illness. This is especially true for people who experience life-threatening illness such as cancer or heart disease. Those who heal and go on to enjoy good health and well-being listen within and act on the intuitive healing messages that they receive. Intuition connects us to the wisdom of our physical body and to the forces of healing.

Like Teresa, more and more conventional physicians see the value and participate in what was once viewed as unorthodox and even unusual types of healing modalities. When medical professionals started to send me clients and book sessions with me, I realized that the value of intuitive energy health information was becoming undeniable.

The medical world is rapidly changing. Alternative therapies and treatments are being integrated into conventional settings. This evolution in health care is in part being fueled by individuals who are taking back their power. We are increasingly becoming aware of how our emotions, thoughts, attitudes, diet, spirituality, and daily choices affect our health and well-being. With this awareness we become empowered to heal and create better health by intuitively listening to the needs of our physical body, healing our inner emotional wounds, changing our thoughts and beliefs, and embracing the power of our spirit.

Your Body Is Always Communicating

Although I am now confident in my ability to accurately intuit health energy information, I was initially apprehensive about asserting myself in this area. The domain of health, healing, and illness seemed to belong to those in the conventional medical field, but I have long since realized that intuitive health awareness is everyone's birthright. We all have within us the innate power to intuit energy information and experience optimum health and well-being.

In the medical intuition classes I teach I have found that others are also somewhat hesitant to harness their intuition for health and healing. We tend to view health information as the domain of the conventional medical community. Many shy away from developing their ability in this area. Yet, the physical body is wise and communicative. It is always speaking to us and everyone can become a better listener. The physical and subtle energies of the body are like a diary that contains all that you have ever experienced, thought, and felt. You can learn how to use and develop your natural intuition to tap into this treasure of energy information for yourself and for others. Developing your intuitive ability will also enable you to make informed and wise health care decisions and choose the best health care professionals for your specific needs.

You are Intuitive

Your rational thinking self may question and doubt that you have the ability to tune in to the complexity of the physical body and all of its intricacies and intuit correct and helpful health information and guidance. Yet, there is a part of you that lies underneath the rational and logical mind that is naturally intuitive and can access, receive, and interpret the important and useful mind, body, and spirit energy information that is constantly broadcast your way.

Intuition is your most natural wisdom. It is always present. Although everyone is intuitive, many people disregard their natural intuitive tendencies because they have a preconceived idea of what it means to be psychic or intuitive. If they do not receive visions of future events or visually see loved ones on the other side or know what is going to happen in the future, they assume they are not intuitive. When it comes to our ability to use our intuition in the area of health and wellness we often react in a similar way. Many have a preconceived idea that the ability to intuit health energy information is a rare talent that only a few possess, but whether your interest is to use your intuition to tune in to your own health or to help and be of service to others as well, you already have within you this innate intuitive sense.

In my book *Discover Your Psychic Type* I describe the four basic ways our intuition naturally surfaces. My books *Love and Intuition* and *You Are a Medium* offer a similar approach of understanding and exploring your natural intuitive type to develop and effectively use your intuition. You may primarily intuit through your emotions, your thoughts, or you may absorb energy information into your physical body or your energy field. This book will teach you how to recognize the way you naturally intuit and how to effectively develop these innate abilities into practical and useful medical intuitive skills.

Medical intuition encompasses a broad range of intuitive abilities and possibilities. The core of medical intuition is the ability to intuitively tune in to the organs and the cardiovascular, skeletal, glandular, and other systems of the body and identify imbalance, disease, or dysfunction. Medical intuitives are also often able to decipher the ignored and hidden emotional, psychological, personality, and spiritual influences that are creating illness and preventing healing.

How to Use This Book

The first steps of this journey of health and wellness begin with taking a quiz to become more aware of your energy health. Through easy-to-follow exercises you will then learn how to identify when you are absorbing and overloaded with detrimental energy and how to improve and heal your physical, mental, emotional, and spiritual energy health. Good energy health is a vital component to developing your intuition.

The next section includes a quiz to help you to determine the specific way you are already intuiting health energy information. Understanding your innate medical intuitive type will enable and encourage you to hone in on the area of health and wellness where you can have the most impact and experience the best results.

There will be certain areas of medical intuition where you will naturally excel and other areas that may take more time to develop and refine. For instance, you may choose to focus on and develop expertise in the ability to intuitively tune in to disease and illness in the physical body, or you may find that you are more interested in intuiting the spiritual, emotional, and mental influences and imbalances that contribute to both illness and healing.

Along with better understanding of your innate medical intuition type, this section also introduces the five basic medical intuitive skills. You will learn about the psychic skills of clairvoyance, which is the ability to see and perceive energy information; clairsentience, the ability to feel and sense energy; clairaudience, the ability to intuitively hear energy information; claircognizance, which is clear intuitive knowing; and vibrational sensitivity, the ability to sense and understand energy vibration.

In the next section you will also explore the subtle energy body, which is comprised of the aura or energy field, the chakras, and the meridians. These energies disclose past and present emotional, mental, and spiritual patterns and provide important insight into why we become ill and how to heal. Using the five medical intuitive skills, you will learn and practice how to intuitively tune in to the subtle energy body—the pulsating and colorful network of energy that surrounds our physical body—and discover its connection to past, present, and future disease and illness.

The next section shows you how to tune in to your own health and well-being through easy-to-follow exercises. As your confidence as a medical intuitive increases, you may want to share this ability with others.

In this book, through a step-by-step process, you will learn how to intuitively tune in to another's health and how to effectively communicate and correctly interpret what you receive. Other important areas of medical intuition, such as the ethics of medical intuition, the importance of maintaining healthy boundaries, and what to do when you are wrong are also discussed. You will also learn how your dreams and synchronicities inform and guide you to better health and healing, how to enlist the support of your spirit helpers, and how to discover the natural healing gifts of your intuitive type.

Your Path to Health

Both extraordinary and practical, developing medical intuition is an effective path to actualizing your utmost potential in mind, body, spirit, health, and well-being. Developing your natural ability to intuitively tune in to the energy body, access health information, and positively influence your and others' health, is transformative. Good health and wellness is a state of being that is more than simply a lack of pain or illness. It is an enlightened perspective and the activation of your inner power to work in harmony with beneficial healing forces to create the best life possible.

I invite you to take part in this exciting intuitive adventure into the mind, body, and spirit. I hope to offer you a unique perspective and intuitive tools that will enlighten, inspire, and empower you on your journey into the awe-inspiring realm of intuition and health.

Section 1

MEDICAL
INTUITION PREP

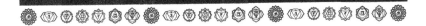

1

KEYS TO UNLOCKING THE MEDICAL INTUITIVE WITHIN YOU

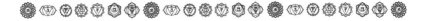

Medical intuition is the ability to intuit health energy information without reliance on an external source. The idea of medicine and intuition joining forces and harmoniously working together to heal and care for the physical body may seem unlikely. The logical scientific world of medicine and the mystical realm of intuition appear to be at opposite ends of the spectrum. Yet, conventional medicine and intuition share common roots.

Early humans looked to the cosmos and the gods for healing and good health. In ancient Greece, Asclepius was the god of medicine. He was believed to have been raised by Apollo and taught the art of healing. The ill and suffering went to temples erected in his honor. It is said that Hippocrates, the legendary "father of medicine," may have begun his career in one of these temples. In these holy sanctuaries, the sick and suffering would report their dreams or visions to a priest who would interpret them and then prescribe the appropriate treatment based on his interpretation. In the indigenous pre-modern world, and still today in many areas, people seek help and healing through the intervention of a shaman. Shamans influence, interact, and elicit healing intervention for the needy from the spirit world. They heal by entering into an altered state of consciousness where they become aware of the wounds, illnesses, and emotional, physical, and mental dysfunctions of an individual. Healing is achieved by bringing balance and wholeness to the soul and spirit of those who suffer.

Early Medical Intuitives

In the modern Western world, the practice of using intuition for medical information dates back to Phineas Parkhurst Quimby, who began an intuitive healing practice in 1854. Quimby was a philosopher, magnetizer, mesmerist, healer, and inventor who worked and lived in Portland, Maine. He believed the intuitive mind held the answers to the origin of disease and illness and how to promote healing and restoration. Known as the sleeping prophet, Edgar Cayce (1877–1945) may be the most widely recognized medical intuitive. As a young man he lost his voice while ill. During a hypnosis session he described in detail the reason for his paralyzed vocal chords and the cure. Once awake, the remedy he spoke of while in trance was administered and his voice returned. Soon after, Cayce discovered that in this sleeplike trance state he was able to access accurate and helpful health and other information for clients. There are over fourteen thousand of his recorded readings, most of which centered on health and well-being. In 1987, Dr. Norm Shealy and Caroline Myss popularized the term "medical intuitive." Dr. Shealy conducted research on the use of intuition in medical practice with Caroline Myss, who was able to accurately describe illness in others.

Medical intuition involves more than intuitively examining and diagnosing the physical body. It encompasses a holistic perspective of the connection and interaction of the body, mind, and spirit. Concerned with an integrated sensitivity to one's overall well-being, medical intuitives provide useful and often surprising energy information that may not always fit within the parameters of conventional medicine. Medical intuitives believe that dynamic health and well-being is more than the healthy functioning of the physical body. Instead, it is within the emotional, mental, and spiritual energy influences that true health emerges.

Approaching Health and Intuition

The decision to develop medical intuition is a bold act. Both the scientific medical world and the unseen realm of intuition can at times be intimidating. Claiming your innate ability to intuitively tune in to your health is a taking back of your personal power.

For many, the healthcare system is like a maze, challenging and confusing to maneuver through. When we are ill or in pain the array of choices in doctors, health care professionals, and conventional and alternative medical options can be overwhelming. Over time the scientific and medical community has overtaken our confidence in our ability to trust our decision making. Given the years of study and the financial resources that go into becoming a health care provider, it is no surprise that we leave our health needs to the care of professionals. Yet, for all of the medical research and astronomical amount of money that goes into understanding the complexity of illness, disease, and how to cure and heal the body, many people still suffer and do not heal.

To maintain good health and heal illness and disease requires a transformative attitude and positive participation. Medical intuition tunes in to the unseen and often unknown influences that affect health. Once these influences are revealed it then becomes possible to confront and heal the imbalances and issues that are at the root of illness. Medical intuition empowers us to make informed medical choices and activate our inner healing forces to create good health in body, mind, and spirit.

Spontaneous Intuitive Health Messages

For some, intuition may seem to be an untrustworthy and mystical gift that only a few can fully grasp and effectively utilize. Unlike science and medicine, intuition is associated with the hidden, mysterious, and esoteric realm. Yet, we are all intuitive and every day we listen and act on our inner knowing in various ways. For example, you may trust an intuitive hunch and call a friend or family member that you sense may be in need. Upon first meeting another you might listen to a persistent inner voice that tells you to be careful. When confronted with having to make a choice in a job or career you might pick the one that you most intuitively feel will work out, despite a lack of logical validation. In the same way you may receive spontaneous intuitive messages about your health or the health of others.

Your body is wise and always communicating with you. For instance, Jennifer is a thirty-nine-year-old account executive I recently gave a medical intuitive reading to. When I began the session I could feel itching and bumpy inflammation on her skin. I told her of my immediate intuitive findings and she confirmed that she had come to see me for insight into a rash that would not go away. She had already been to her doctor and a dermatologist. While she got temporary relief from medication, the rash always returned.

"I want to know the cause of this rash," she told me.

"I keep seeing an image of bright red strawberries," I answered.

"I had a feeling it was the strawberries," she excitedly said. "I have been eating them like crazy this past spring and summer. I woke up one morning and heard an inner voice telling me that my rash was caused by eating too many strawberries. I asked my doctor about it, but he wasn't sure this was the problem. "

I continued explaining what I was intuiting to Jennifer, "I'm also feeling frustration or aggravation with work. An issue with your job is stressing your system."

"I'm not surprised. I've had a feeling that the frustration I've been feeling at work may be affecting my rash too. I was moved a few months ago to another department at work. I didn't get a raise and I've been overwhelmed. They never asked me if I wanted a new job. One day I was just told to go work with another group. It has been aggravating."

Jennifer, like many of my clients, already had an intuitive awareness of the influences affecting her health. I simply provided her with confirmation on what she intuitively already knew. Once she better understood these issues she took the needed actions to heal her rash.

Not only do we quite naturally intuit the influences that affect our health, we also spontaneously intuit the health of others. This is what happened to Kevin, a curly-headed young man of nineteen. Kevin came into my office and quietly sat down on the couch.

"I don't know exactly why I'm here," he explained. "My mother told me about a session she had with you few years ago and I thought maybe you could help me. "

"Would you like a reading?" I asked.

"Maybe ... yes ... I didn't really come here for me," he hesitantly began. "I think my mother is sick. I have a feeling that something is wrong. I don't know what. But I just know that something is wrong. I can't explain it. I look at her and something feels off. I don't know if I'm crazy or having an anxiety attack. Can you tell if my mother is ill?"

"Does your mother know that you came to see me? She would have to give her consent for me to look at her health," I told Kevin.

"Oh yes, she gave me your information to set up an appointment. I asked her to go to the doctor and she did. But this feeling will not go away. My mom knows I'm here. She thought maybe you can help me and her if necessary." Kevin looked anxious and understandably nervous.

When I remotely scanned Kevin's mother's body, I was drawn to her lower abdomen. I paused in this area to collect more energy information and quickly felt and saw a dark heaviness in her upper colon. The dark area was dense and I knew that it was a tumor and that she needed immediate medical attention.

"You said your mom went to her doctor for a checkup?" I asked Kevin.

"That's what she said. It was several months ago, maybe six or more," he explained.

I did not want to further alarm Kevin, but I confirmed his intuitive suspicions. "Your mom needs to go to a doctor. The sooner the better," I told him. "Would you have her call me? I can explain more to her."

"Is it serious? What's wrong?" Kevin interrupted me.

"There's a problem in her colon," I informed him. "You're not crazy or having an anxiety attack. Your intuition is spot on. Your mom is fortunate that you listened to your intuition."

A few hours after Kevin left, I heard from his mother. I explained to her what my scan of her body revealed. Several weeks later I received another call from her letting me know that she was currently recovering from surgery.

"I would like to schedule a session. I need to understand the causes of the cancer. I have a feeling that this is about more than just my physical health. There are some emotional and past issues I need to explore. Maybe my son's intuition is rubbing off on me, but I know that I have some work to do to fully heal," she said.

Like Kevin, we have all at one time or another most likely experienced a persistent feeling or sensed that something was just not right with our health or someone else's. When we ignore and deny these intuitive impulses, we usually later regret it.

Transformation of Thought and Belief

Behind spontaneous episodes of intuitive health awareness lays a potent innate ability that everyone possesses. Successfully developing medical intuition involves more than simply learning a new skill. When you make the decision to harness your innate intuition you set in motion a journey of spiritual growth and increased self-awareness. It will likely challenge you to redefine your view of reality and what you are capable of.

Activating your intuition begins with releasing your self-imposed limitations and trusting an inner force of awareness. If you are questioning that there exists within you a wise inner knower, you are not alone. Before I begin teaching an introductory intuition class, there is usually an uneasy restlessness that circulates around the room. After I introduce myself, I explain the basics of intuition development. Then, as soon as possible, I start an intuitive exercise. There is a detectable sigh of relief and shift in the room once everyone begins to turn on their intuitive sensors. This is especially true of developing medical intuition. As much as we desire to intuitively tune in to our health and be of service to others with their health concerns, doubt and the fear of being incorrect and unable to access any useful information often surfaces. This stress can unfortunately cripple our efforts at accessing our intuitive knowing.

In general, people approach developing medical intuition with a little more trepidation than they do other types of intuitive development. Most people in the intuitive classes I teach eagerly attempt to contact their loved ones on the other side or intuit insights about a love relationship or career prospects, but the idea of intuiting health information can provoke tremors of doubt and uncertainty.

There are understandable reasons for this. When it comes to health concerns we are accustomed to seeking the advice and recommendations of knowledgeable professionals. Almost daily in the news we learn of new discoveries in research and advancements in understanding and treating illness and disease. Health care is a multibillion dollar industry, driving the economies of countries all over the world. The quiet voice of intuition can seem a small and insignificant contender in the health care enterprise.

Yet, the body is an intuitive goldmine. It wants to be heard and is always speaking to us. Your spirit knows what you need in order to physically, emotionally, and mentally heal and thrive. Nature has equipped us with the ability to tune in to this wisdom through our natural intuition. In addition to providing you with an in-depth and comprehensive view of your health, medical intuition enhances your awareness and interaction with conventional and alternative medicine providers and services. It offers you a personal and insightful view of your health and well-being that empowers you to make conscious choices and decisions. Medical intuition is not in conflict with conventional and alternative medical care. Instead it informs you as to what you most need in order to heal and enables you to make choices that support your highest good.

Informing, Not Diagnosing

Medical intuition is the intuitive art of receiving and interpreting energy information in the area of health and wellness. Unlike physicians who diagnose illness and disease and prescribe medication and other medical treatments, medical intuitives inform but do not diagnose. When working with others, your primary role as a medical intuitive is intuitively tuning in to and interpreting energy information. One of the biggest challenges for the beginning medical intuitive is to resist prematurely labeling and diagnosing an intuitively detected dysfunction and imbalance. You are not working within the conventional medical paradigm. Instead, the paradigm for medical intuition is inclusive and holistic. The parameters are much broader than those of the conventional medical community.

For a medical intuitive, physical health is influenced by many factors from both the unseen realm of essence and from the tangible material world. Your physical body, the vibrancy of your subtle energy, your connection to your spirit, and your emotional and mental energies are all considered. A medical intuitive's role does not stop once a dysfunction is detected in the physical body. Intuitively tuning in to the underlying energetic causes behind physical problems and listening to the wisdom of the mind, body, and spirit are just as important.

Trusting Your Intuition

As a medical intuitive you are assisted by cosmic and divine forces. When you intuit for the highest good for self and others you never work alone. There are spiritual forces that guide and benevolently support you in your efforts. Your job is to align with these forces and open yourself as a channel of wisdom, love, and healing for others and for yourself. It is always a temptation with medical intuitive work for the ego to take over and attempt to control an intuitive session.

Although a background in science, medicine, and anatomy can be helpful in effectively intuiting the health of the body, it is not necessary. Not having a medical background allows you to depend exclusively on your intuition. This can be a blessing. It has been when I have felt most challenged that I have most readily sought and accepted the help of higher forces. This has always paid off for me. When I teach medical intuition, I primarily teach how to intuitively read the human energy field.

The Basics

Developing medical intuition is in many ways similar to developing intuitive abilities for use in other areas. Here are a few basics to remember as you proceed.

You are naturally intuitive

Everyone is intuitive, including you. Just as everyone can sing, some of us might need to take voice lessons to refine natural talent. So it is with intuition. Although you have innate intuitive ability you may need to further develop it to make the most of this useful innate sense.

Your intuition is the voice of your spirit

Your intuition emerges from the depth of your spirit. Connected to the source of all that is, your spirit is eternal energy and has access to all wisdom and perfect love. It communicates to you through your intuition.

Your physical body is energy

Your body is a dense form of energy. Despite its appearance as a solid mass, you are particles of vibrating energy.

Your intuition operates outside of time and space

Intuition is not restricted by the laws of the material world. It is your window to a realm flowing with unlimited possibilities. When you tap into your intuition you work outside of the confines of the physical and finite.

You have access to the wisdom and love of the universe; you can personally rely on this power to assist you as a medical intuitive

You may feel alone in a world of random events. Yet, you are known, loved, and supported in a personal way. This may make no sense to logical reasoning. Don't give your power to the overthinking mind. An invisible presence assists you.

You can communicate with energy

We tend to think of energy as an unconscious and detached force. Yet, energy is alive and responsive. It is interactive and will respond and reply to your requests. Medical intuition is an interactive dialogue with energy. The body, emotions, thoughts, and your spirit are comprised of energy with which you can communicate.

Have a clear intent

Energy responds to your request and intent. Although the voice of the ego may bombard you with distracting thoughts and emotions, put your intent into words and be determined to access energy information for the highest good. During a medical intuitive body scan keep your intent simple. As you move through the many different aspects and areas of the body you can stay focused by saying such things as: "Show me an image of the sinuses." Or "How is the grief and loss I feel affecting me physically?"

Trust your first impression

Although I encourage you to take your time and not rush to conclusions and judgments, it is important to pay attention to your first intuitive impression. Observe what you initially receive and give it space to continue to develop and speak to you.

Use your imagination

Your imagination and intuition work together. Imagination translates intuitive energy information into a form that you can decipher and better understand. Although there are times when you may come across illusory images that are not connected to your intuition, for the most part during intuitive work your imagination is working in unison with your intuition. In time you will be able to detect when the images you perceive are representative of energy information and when they have no corresponding energetic influence.

Take a leap

At some point during every intuitive reading you will feel as if you are jumping off the abyss of the known and into the unknown. Resist the temptation to play it safe. Your development will not progress unless you allow yourself to enter into the fuzzy and risky area of the unfamiliar. This is where it all happens.

Doubt is common, let it go

Doubt is one of the biggest stumbling blocks to intuitive development. Its normal, so don't let it limit and control you. That nagging voice that tells you that you are about to make a fool of yourself, that you are no good at intuitive insight, and that it is best to pack it up and go do something else will likely hound you. This is the ego attempting to gain control of the situation. Intuitive insight springs from the soul. The voice of doubt does not have to cripple you.

It is okay to be wrong

Everyone wants to be intuitively correct, right, genius, and spot on. The truth of the matter is that unless you allow yourself to make mistakes and misinterpret or misidentify energy information you will not progress very far. It is as important to be wrong as it is to be right when developing your intuition. In time, you recognize when and why you are misreading or misinterpreting energy information and the intuitive feel of when you are correct.

Communicate what you receive

Describe the energy that you intuitively perceive as authentically and accurately as possible. Do not attempt to use medical terms and fit what you intuit into a neat and logical package. At first you may fumble for words and feel as if what you are describing makes no sense. Eventually the right and left brain will work together to form a cohesive understanding. As the right brain receives the intuitive impulses, the left brain will connect the correct interpretation and words to the energy information. You eventually will become more trusting and confident in the spontaneous language that emerges to describe what you are intuiting.

Practice

It is helpful to practice intuitive skills as much as possible. One of the obstacles of developing medical intuition is the availability of subjects. If you have family and friends with whom you would like to practice your intuitive skills, be sure to get their permission before you intuitively tune in to their energy. It is not ethical to intuitively read anyone's physical body without their permission.

However, there are other avenues you can explore to practice your skills. Every living being has an energy field. You can learn quite a bit from the energy field of plants and trees and even rocks. All living things will communicate to you. Animals are also wonderful practice subjects. Your pets will love it when you tune in to their energy. Your pets are quite psychic and are aware of when you intuitively communicate with them. As an added benefit you will be able to address any unknown health issues they may have.

You can also practice on birds and squirrels and any other animal that you cross paths with. They may be a little more challenging as they tend to come and go quite quickly. Yet, I have had surprising insights from intuiting the energy of animals and plants. All living beings have consciousness, thoughts, emotions, and spirits.

Keep these guidelines in mind as you progress through the material in this book. With this intuitive development preparation and foundation you are now ready to tune in to the innate intuitive energy of your body, mind, and spirit.

2

YOUR
ENERGY HEALTH

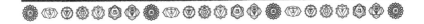

I envision a time when health care and wellness not only includes our physical, mental, and emotional health but our energy health as well. Good energy health supports, enhances, and promotes a healthy mind, body, and spirit. Intuitive awareness is a conscious relationship to energy. To more quickly develop your intuition and become a clear and accurate medical intuitive, it is necessary to become conscious of the way that you unknowingly absorb and connect and relate to energy.

Even if you do not consider yourself a proficient intuitive, you are absorbing the energy of your friends, family, and coworkers on a daily basis. Not only do you soak in the energy of those in your immediate environment, you are also likely absorbing the energy of distant events and the thoughts and feelings of those miles and miles away. In this age of the Internet and social media, we are more exposed than ever to events that take place across the globe. We have an intimate window into what others are feeling, their beliefs, and their struggles. This increases our intuitive vulnerability to sympathetically absorb the energy of that which touches our hearts or causes us distress and concern. Energy is not restricted to time and place. It knows no physical boundaries and it is always present.

Developing your ability to better communicate and work with energy increases your intuitive sensitivity. As we collectively become more aware of the power of intuition and energy dynamics, the reality of our oneness with all others becomes more apparent. This awareness helps us to understand the influences that our thoughts, emotions, beliefs, and spiritual consciousness have on our health and well-being and the health of others near and far. Just as we absorb the energy of others, they absorb our energy. We are each individually, either positively or negatively, contributing to the collective whole. In the not-too-distant future, we will know ourselves more as energy beings than physical beings.

Health Care of the Future

Medical intuition and energy medicine is the health care of the future. Now is the time to become more aware of your energy health. As Albert Einstein taught us, energy is indestructible. It cannot be created nor destroyed. It simply changes form. At physical death your energy self lives on. Energy exists beyond the confines of time and space and is more powerful than the physical body. When you activate and harness your energetic vibrational power you can heal, restore, and sustain your physical body, your emotions, and your mental health.

Many of the people I work with as a medical intuitive have poor energy health. They may be overburdened with toxins and negativity or energetically out of balance due to absorbed environmental and harmful energy. Good physical, mental, and emotional health begins with a strong energetic constitution. Disturbances and toxins in the energy body are at the root of many illnesses, chronic physical pain, emotional imbalances, and mental disorders. Once energy comes into balance and positive energy replaces toxic and stagnant energy, the body responds and heals. A healthy energy body also reduces emotional and mental stress and anxiety, insomnia, and exhaustion, and restores endocrine system health, balances our hormones, allows us to lose weight, and restores the muscular and skeletal system.

The following quiz will help you to identify the quality of your energy health.

Quiz: Energy Health Indicator			
	Often 3 pts.	Sometimes 2 pts.	Never/ Rarely 1 pt.
1. I get headaches from bright lights or fluorescent lighting.			
2. I am apathetic and uninterested in many things.			
3. I wake up at night feeling intense emotions.			
4. I am forgetful and I am often late.			
5. I have no appetite; food does not appeal to me.			
6. I am preoccupied with random ideas, inventions, solutions, but I have no way to implement them.			
7. I am disconnected from my family and friends. I feel like a stranger in this world.			
8. I sleep too much and feel lethargic.			
9. I overeat, especially sweets and carbohydrates.			
10. I experience energy surges and a racing heart.			
11. I don't know why I am on this earth; I want to go home.			

Quiz: Energy Health Indicator (cont.)	Often 3 pts.	Sometimes 2 pts.	Never/ Rarely 1 pt.
12. I have insomnia.			
13. I spend a lot of time daydreaming and fantasizing.			
14. I experience persistent headaches.			
15. I have premonitions of doom or disasters.			
16. I have chronic allergies.			
17. I see dark spots and lines of energy in the air.			
18. I want to flee my current situation.			
19. I experience overwhelming feelings and emotions.			
20. I experience uncontrolled psychic knowing.			
21. I am very clumsy.			
22. I have chronic negative thoughts.			
23. I have chronic itchy skin and unexplained rashes.			
24. I am sensitive and can be easily hurt by others' thoughts and feelings toward me.			
25. My dreams disturb my sleep.			
26. I experience sudden feelings of panic and/or fear.			

Quiz: Energy Health Indicator (cont.)			
	Often 3 pts.	Sometimes 2 pts.	Never/ Rarely 1 pt.
27. No matter how much I sleep I am exhausted.			
28. I experience free-floating anxiety.			
29. I have digestive problems and chronic upset stomach.			
30. I feel that the mundane world is boring and meaningless.			
31. I am often spacy and confused.			
32. I have unexplained weight gain.			
33. I have intense spiritual experiences followed by bouts of depression.			
34. I see or feel the presence of agitating ghosts or spirits.			
35. I have uncontrolled emotional mood swings.			
36. I experience unexplained body aches and pains.			
37. My mind races and I cannot focus.			
38. I can go and go all day; I have unlimited energy. It is hard for me to relax and slow down.			
39. I hear negative and fear-producing inner voices.			
40. I have out-of-body experiences that are out of my control.			

Quiz: Energy Health Indicator (cont.)			
	Often 3 pts.	Sometimes 2 pts.	Never/ Rarely 1 pt.
41. I experience past life interruptions.			
42. Negative spirits and ETs attempt to get my attention.			
Add Scores			

If your totals equal between:

101–129 = A

68–100 = B

42–67 = C

A. ENERGY BOTTOM FEEDER

You are absorbing lower vibration and possibly toxic energy. This is unhealthy for your mind, body, and spirit. Steps need to be taken to come into energetic balance. It is important to learn how to protect yourself from being bombarded with energy that is not in your highest good.

B. WALKING THE ENERGY TIGHTROPE

You are on the precipice of being overwhelmed by harmful energy. You are experiencing moments of dipping into the cesspool of lower vibrations. It is important that you learn how to discern energy that is in your highest good from energy vibrations that drain your reserves. By becoming more sensitive to the quality of the energy in your environment and what you are absorbing, you can come into balance and increase your positive energy bank.

C. THE AXIS OF HARMONY

You are not showing signs of being overwhelmed by negative and toxic energy. You can choose to further open to the higher vibrations and increase the flow of positive energy into your body, mind, and spirit.

Continue to stay aware and trust your intuitive sense of your energy environment. You are most likely the person that everyone wants to be close to. Others feel positive, uplifted, and light just being next to you.

Creating Good Energy Health

The following steps will help you to heal, improve, and create and sustain good energy health.

As you refine and improve your intuitive skills and abilities you develop more sensitivity to energy vibration and essence. It becomes vitally important for you to be alert and mindful of your daily interaction with energy. We do not absorb negative, fear-based, and toxic energy because we want to. Most people unknowingly and without conscious intent absorb the pain, stress, negative thoughts, fear, and anger of others and the world. Just as unknowingly eating food or drinking water that is unclean or contaminated will cause illness and infection, absorbing low-vibration energy affects you even when you are unaware of it. The following steps will help you to heal, improve, and create and sustain good energy health.

The first step to establishing energetic balance and attracting positive energy is to activate the power of your spirit and take charge of your life. You can regulate and control what you absorb and interact with. Your spirit is the eternal part of you that is connected to the highest vibrations of love and wisdom. As your conscious personality self comes into alignment with your spirit, you act as one force of unified power. You attract and unite with the positive. The dark, negative, and dysfunctional is repelled.

Your spirit speaks to you through your intuition. On a daily basis your intuition can guide you toward those situations, activities, thoughts, emotions, and environments that uplift and increase your positive energy quota. Every day you knowingly and unknowingly make choices that either promote good energy health or add an energetic burden to your body, mind, and emotions. Your intuition can steer you away from people who have ill intent and those who drain your energy or try to energetically unload their negativity or stress on you. It can help you to avoid dangerous situations and instead point you in the direction of those circumstances that fill you with love and strengthen you. Your intuition can help you know the source of what is exhausting and depleting your energy reserves and adversely affecting your mind, body, and spirit.

Intuitive guidance is usually quite simple and straightforward. Listen to your body. Pay attention to what stimulates queasy, uneasy, gut feelings of stress and dread, nervousness, and tension. Your body does not lie. Feel your emotions. Notice what fills you with dread, or provokes anxiety, fear, stress, and apprehension. Pay attention to negative self-talk and the inner voice that tells you that something is "off" or "not right." When you get an intuitive flash of danger or a warning, do not override it with overly logical arguments. Remember your dreams and work to decipher their message. Your intuition will often work through your dreams to bring to light what your conscious mind is denying. When you experience any of these intuitive messages, take some time alone and ask within for more guidance and a better understanding.

Remember that appearances are deceiving. Be willing to explore the energy of all that you come into contact with, both near and far.

You Are Love

Love is our most powerful source of high vibration energy. When you love yourself and others, and treat yourself and others with respect, then protective, healing, and revitalizing energy flows through you. Know who you are. You are love incarnate in a world of material matter. Loving yourself is not an ego event. Instead, it is the honoring and remembrance of who you are. When you love yourself you are reminding yourself of your true spiritual nature. You are saying: *I am one with love.*

In the same way that you are love, so is everyone that you meet. Connect with the most loving and positive energy within others. Many loving people who wish to help others tend to absorb others' emotional sadness, pain, or stress in a misguided attempt to heal and help them.

When people show you their emotional helplessness, wounds, and their lack of self-awareness, do not let this fool you. They are as connected to the eternal source of love and wisdom as you are. What resides within you, resides within them. Have compassion and treat others with kindness, but do not identify with their wounds and victimization. When you focus on another's misfortune or helplessness, you only make it stronger and blind them from their true essence. Be the one who takes the blinders off. Love others in the highest sense by seeing the power within them to experience perfect love and peace.

Behind all of the discord, emotional trauma, and pain that we experience, a perfect healing and restorative love waits for our acknowledgement. When you see this within yourself you can see it within another. A great power resides within each one of us, even when appearances seem to be showing us the opposite. See the light in others and they will see it in themselves.

EXERCISE: EMOTIONAL CLEARING

- If you feel that you have absorbed toxic emotional energy, like pain, anger, and grief from another, this exercise will help you to clear your energy field.

- Take a long deep breath. Breathe and relax and allow your emotions to surface. Begin by putting words to your emotions. It sounds simple, but we rarely identify how we feel and the source of our feelings.

- Focus on one emotion at a time. Ask yourself if the source of this feeling is within you or if you have absorbed this feeling from an outside source.

- Take a moment and breathe a few long, deep, cleansing breaths. Listen within. You will soon have a sense of whether or not you have generated this feeling or if you have absorbed it from another. Trust your initial intuitive response.

- If you intuit that this is a feeling that you have absorbed from an outer source, intend to let it go. You do not need to know who or where it came from. Simply breathe and affirm within that you are releasing what is not yours.

- If this is a self-generated emotion, ask within for guidance as to what you need in order to heal or transform. Give the emotion a voice and listen to it.

- This may be a long or short process. If you need help in re-solving and understanding how to emotionally heal, ask for the advice or counsel of someone who you trust or a therapist.

- At times we absorb others' emotional energy and this triggers a similar emotion with both people. You may need to both release and heal discordant emotions.

Love is the most powerful and health-promoting energy here and in the unseen realms. Whatever you are feeling that does not vibrate to the energy of love is an energy drain on your system. At your core, you are love. It is always within you. Love can help heal your physical body and empower you to experience the goodness in all of life, no matter what your current circumstances may be. Release your anger and grievances, and forgive yourself and others. Every day acknowledge and express gratitude for all of the good in your life. Open your heart, and call forth the love within. Let it move through you and invigorate and restore your body, mind, and spirit.

The Power of Thought Energy

Although we like to think that our thoughts are original and personal, this is not always the case. There is collective thought energy that we all tap into. You may be unknowingly affected by the thoughts of others near and far away. Thoughts are energy and they travel from one individual to the next, influencing and affecting people across the globe.

From a young age we are overtly and covertly taught to accept the beliefs, biases, ideas, and judgments of others. There are many ways throughout your day that you are exposed to and absorb negative thought energy. People often bond to one another through common dislikes, negative opinions, grievances, and aversions. From political opinions to cultural beliefs about behavior, to the judgments and ignorance we harbor about other nationalities and religions and sexual orientations, there is an appealing security in identifying with group mentality. To belong feels safe. Many feel that it is necessary to support and accept the thought energy of their workplace and coworkers in order to make a living and thrive in their career. We compromise our inner truth and stifle the still voice of our spirit in order to live in a world that seems to have power over us. Our fear motivates us to automatically and unconsciously accept negative thought energy and make it our own. This blind allegiance leads us away from our most true and powerful self.

You are not your opinions, your beliefs, your thoughts, and your judgments. You are spirit energy connected to the source of all love and wisdom. When you accept thought energy that does not vibrate to your core spirit you add an energetic burden to your body, mind, and spirit. You become confused, stressed, anxious, and eventually ill.

Like love, the authentic inner self can never be tarnished or destroyed, and it can never leave you. It is always a source of strength and healing. As you develop intuitive sensitivity you begin to hear and listen to its ever-present inner voice. We all have some degree of negative thought energy. The good news is that everyone has the innate ability to release it and bond to their powerful authentic self.

Many fear that they will be lonely and considered odd if they live their truth. This will not happen. Instead, when you know who you are and are in integrity with your truth, you emit an infectious and magnetic ray of light. Others are attracted to the invisible core of your power and strength. They sense and experience their own power in your presence. By your willingness to be authentically you, you empower others to live in their truth.

EXERCISE: RELEASE AND TRANSFORM THOUGHT ENERGY

Become aware of the thoughts, beliefs, judgments, and ideas that are not your personal truth. You can begin in this way:

- Take a long, deep breath and exhale. Continue to breathe and relax and listen within. As you do this you will likely become aware of two opposing energies. Listen to both of them. Do not dismiss or stuff away either one.

- The origin of some of your thoughts is your ego. These are the thoughts that you have absorbed from others and the collective ego mind. You will recognize them because they will likely be critical, demeaning, judgmental, and negative. They may try to persuade you to stop this exercise. Say one of these thoughts aloud.

- As you say this thought feel the energy of your body. Does it feel weakened, tired, tense, depleted, or anxious?

- Now ask for a thought from your authentic self. Allow it to emerge from the inner depth of your spirit. Say it aloud. Feel the energy of your body. Does this thought calm you, give you energy, relax and strengthen you? Original thought is always positive and wise as it springs from source energy. It is unencumbered with judgment, bias, fear, and negativity.

- Continue to listen to your thoughts. Those thoughts that weaken you can be released and let go of. Simply say the thought, breathe, and release it. You no longer need this thought. Ask that it be sent into the light of wisdom and love to be transformed into positive energy.

- Ask for the thoughts of truth to fill you. Listen to these thoughts and allow them to move through you, invigorating and healing you.

Every day, without being aware of it, we either accept or reject the thought energy that comes our way. Some of our thoughts come from external sources and other thoughts come to us from our inner source of truth. Intend to listen within and absorb the healing thoughts of truth. Your mind, body, and spirit will be restored and become stronger and healthier.

Your Inner Power

Respect yourself and your path in life. We have all come into this world to know who we are. The family that you have been born into, your socioeconomic status, your gender, nationality, and the circumstances and experiences that you confront on a daily basis have been orchestrated to inspire you to come into your most powerful self. Let go of self-blame and guilt. Forgive yourself for those things that you regret and accept each day as a blank page. All of this is temporary. Your situation in life is a role that you have agreed to play in an earth performance that often seems to make no sense. When you respect yourself, others will respect you too. Only accept and expect the best and most positive to come your way.

Embrace your power and know that it is positive energy. Speak your truth. Begin by sharing your opinions with others on significant and not-so-significant issues. Say "yes" when you mean yes and "no" when you mean no.

Your inner power enables you to create and enjoy beauty, abundance, love, well-being, and perfect health. Many people, particularly women, are fearful of acknowledging and claiming their power. They may believe that power is force or ego self-will. In the material world we have misconstrued the true meaning of inner power. Instead of understanding power to be positive source energy we define and experience it as dominance, aggression, authority, and control.

When you do not consciously utilize your power, someone or something will come along and use it for their own purposes. We so easily give our power to others or to something outside of ourselves. When we do this, we become energetically vulnerable and absorb random and often toxic outer vibrations. This creates imbalance in your thoughts, emotions, and your physical body.

Giving Away Power

Every day we unknowingly give away our power in common and deceptive ways. For instance, the friend who has constant drama in her life and needs your advice and help may not be as willing to change as she may seem. She comes to you and expounds on her problems and how others take advantage of her and misunderstand her. You listen and offer words of support and advice. But nothing seems to change. You become increasingly exhausted and feel drained after your encounters with her. Although you would like to help her, your positive energy may only be fueling her need for drama and chaos.

When you look to another for your happiness or believe that you need another's love to heal and make you whole, you are giving away your power. When you feel guilty or uncomfortable around a friend or family member who never gets a lucky break and is envious of your success and happiness, you are giving away your power. If you continually seek the advice of another who you believe knows better than you how to solve your problems and manage your life, you are giving away your power. Many people who are healthy, positive, and loving allow others they feel sorry for or pity to draw energy from them. This is spiritual codependency and eventually leads to feeling drained, exhausted, and ultimately physically ill.

There is a difference between compassion and loving another, and giving away your power. Recognize that the source of the power within you that creates peace, harmony, abundance, and loving relationships in your life is your spirit. When you do this you will begin to recognize that others embody the same power. Your inner power and the inner power of others flows from divine source energy and is unlimited and boundless. Reflect this awareness in your intent and your actions. Resist the temptation to see others as powerless victims. They may not have a conscious awareness of their innate ability to change and transform their current situation. Don't allow this to fool you and compromise your integrity and awareness. Be kind and gentle, loving and compassionate. Yet, always know that despite what others are experiencing, the source of all power is within them as it is within you.

Remind yourself quite often that:

I am connected to the source of all power.
 My power speaks to me through my intuition,
 guiding me to goodness, health, and well-being.

EXERCISE: CALLING BACK YOUR POWER

Your body needs your power to maintain and sustain health and wellness. When you allow others to siphon off your energy, you rob yourself of the necessary fuel for your bodily needs. Energy cords are invisible funnels of energy that extend from you to others. When you give your power away or allow others to draw energy from you, these cords are created. Your energy then moves through these cords to someone or something outside of yourself.

This simple exercise will call back your power.

- Take a long, deep breath. Inhale cleansing breath and exhale any stress and tension. Breathe and relax. Close your eyes and scan your body, starting at the top of the head.

- Set the intent to become aware of any energy cords through which you are either giving your power away or through which you are absorbing others' energy.

- Say and repeat aloud or within yourself: "*I am calling back my power and releasing any energy cords.*"

- As you say this continue to scan your body. Trust your intuition to lead you to where you have an energy cord attachment. You may clairvoyantly see it or feel it as a funnel of vibration being drawn from your body and energy field. When you become aware of a cord ask it: *"What do I need to do in order to release this energy cord?"* Most likely simply having the intent to release it is all that you need to do.

- You may become aware of to whom and where your energy is being funneled, or you may not. If you do know where it is going you may want to ask your angels to heal the imbalance of energy between you and the other person. Then visualize green and gold high-vibration healing energy where the connector had been.

- You do not need to know to whom or where your energy is going. If you come to a cord and are unclear as to its recipient, intend to release it. As you do this, ask for high-vibration healing energy and visualize green and gold energy surrounding the area where the cord was attached.

- Continue to scan your body in this way until all the cords have been released. Visualize yourself surrounded by high-vibration gold, green, and white light. Set the intention to hold your power and love and care for others in a healthy and empowering way.

Intuitive Eating

Food is energy. It is common knowledge that food is an essential part of good health. Most of us from a young age have been taught to eat healthy foods like vegetables, fruit, whole grains, and fish. Yet, our collective diet is full of foods that are overly processed and contain unhealthy fats, too much sugar, and salt. Not only does a poor diet affect your physical body in detrimental ways, it affects your energy health as well. The physical body absorbs necessary vital life force energy from the energy body. If your energy body is weak, the physical body will eventually become weak and out of balance. An unhealthy diet creates a vicious cycle as it weakens both the physical self and the energy body.

Live food has an energy body. Fruit, vegetables, and herbs have an aura. They are energetically comprised of natural elements. They absorb the vibration of the sun, the soil, the rain, and whatever other plant or live being they are close to. Foods like these contribute to our energy health. Not only do they have a high nutritional value, we also strengthen our energy reserves by absorbing their life force energy. Meat, fish, chicken, and dairy products also are live energy foods that have an energy field and aura. They contain animal, fish, or bird vibration and the vibrations that they have been exposed to. Meat that comes from animals, birds, and fish that have been raised in constrictive and oppressive environments will to some extent carry this vibration. For this reason it is best to eat meat, fish, and birds that lived as naturally as possible. Like plants, they carry the vibration of the soil, the sun, the atmosphere, and the live energy that they have consumed.

Processed foods are for the most part energetically inert. They may contain the vibration of the people who work in the plants where they are processed and packaged. To a limited extent they will also carry the positive vibrations of any live food source that they may contain. However, they seldom contain any significant vibrant life force energy. They cannot energetically support you and can detract from your energy health.

Transform Food's Vibration

For many reasons it is always best to eat whole and live foods. However, if this is not possible you can transform the vibration of the food that you eat. Begin by honoring your body and having a conversation with it. Tune in to your physical vibration and lovingly communicate that you are willing to listen to what you need and provide your physical system with high vibration energy. Everything responds to love. Your body will soak in and positively respond to your loving and high vibration intent.

If you do choose to eat processed food, hold it in your hand before you consume it and send it positive energy. Say a prayer and ask for divine presence to be within and surrounding what you are about to eat.

When you eat meat, pause before you consume it and honor the animal, fish, or bird that is providing it to you. Ask the divine presence to be within and surrounding the food that you are about to consume. Send the spirit of the animal gratitude and blessings.

As your intuition increases you will become more sensitive to the energy of food. You will be able to feel a vibrational energy increase or decrease depending on the different foods that you consume. It is likely that you will also become more physically sensitive to what you are eating. Certain foods may begin to disagree with you and you may develop allergies to others. Although this may seem to be detrimental and a sign of poor health, your body may instead be detoxing and better digesting and assimilating what you are eating. As you become more energetically healthy, your body will likely reject lower and negative vibration food and drink. When the energy vibration of your body, mind, and spirit rises into the lofty and transcendent levels of vital life force energy, you will need higher vibration food to maintain this heightened state of being. Trust this process. Listen to your body and allow it to guide you to what it needs. It will likely communicate to you through the physical reactions that you experience with certain foods.

Are You Hungry or Is Your Body Trying to Tell You Something

Your body is a great communicator. Unfortunately we do not always listen and understand its wisdom. Your physical body, your emotions, your thoughts, and your spirit are in constant communication. They are so close and intimate that they essentially operate as one. Western medicine isolates your physical body from your emotions, thoughts, and spirit. If you are in pain or ill, only the physical body is the primary focus. Unfortunately, many people have adopted this same belief and practice. We seldom perceive the many factors and influences that affect our physical health.

Many have an ongoing struggle with weight gain and develop a love/hate attitude with food. For some, it seems that no matter how many diets they try and despite their earnest desire to eat less and lose weight, the scale tips in the opposite direction of this desire. Although we would like to believe that issues with weight are purely diet and exercise related, your thoughts, emotions, and energy field also contribute to weight gain. For many it is necessary to pay attention to these non-physical causes to effectively lose weight.

EXERCISE: EMOTIONAL EATING

Difficult and overwhelming emotions and feelings are some of the most common reasons that people overeat. Intuitively absorbing the negative or stressful emotional energy of others can create inner feelings of restlessness and confusion. Food changes brain chemistry and triggers feel-good emotional and psychological responses. Emotions such as loneliness, anxiousness, sadness, fear, exhaustion, and anger can be uncomfortable. We often reach for food in an attempt to suppress these kinds of feelings and regulate our moods.

Emotions and our desire to eat are powerfully linked. Your intuition can be a valuable tool in helping you to tune in to and balance the underlying emotional energy that leads to weight gain.

- Before you head for the kitchen to satisfy a hunger craving, sit quietly and close your eyes. Take a deep breath and slowly exhale. Continue to breathe deeply and release any stress and tension in your body as you exhale.

- Focus your intuitive awareness within and ask yourself either aloud or silently what you are feeling. Gently repeat this question a few times. Allow any emotions to surface. Put a name to them and continue to breathe and allow as much feeling and emotional energy to surface as possible.

- Listen to the feeling or emotion and dialogue with it. What is it saying to you? Is this your emotional energy or have you intuitively absorbed this from another? Listen and ask what you can do and what you need to heal and calm these emotions and come into a state of inner peace and calm.

- Place your hand on your heart. Breathe in the energy of love and send it from your hand to your heart. Ask for the presence of love and allow it to transform these feelings or release them if they are not yours.

- Continue to breathe long, deep breaths. Take a few moments to feel the presence of healing, unconditional love move through your body.

- Commit to taking care of yourself in a way that will truly satisfy your emotional self. Love yourself. Be kind and compassionate. Let your body know that you are listening and acting in positive ways to take care of yourself.

EXERCISE: INTUITING THE ENERGY OF FOOD

Another useful exercise to do after you have intuitively communicated with your emotions and feelings is to tune in to the energy of the food you are eating. We project a lot of our desires, satisfaction, security, and stress onto food. When you tune in to the energy of what you desire to eat, you discharge food of its projected allure and appeal. You know it for what it is.

- Next time you have a craving or desire to eat, sit quietly and close your eyes. Take a deep breath and slowly exhale. Continue to breathe deeply and release any stress and tension in your body as you exhale.

- Hold some of the food that you desire to eat in your hand. Intuitively tune in to the energy that you associate with this food. Allow all of the thoughts, feelings, and desires that you have projected onto the food to surface. One by one listen to them and realize that this energy has nothing to do with the food you are holding in your hand. When you feel that all of your thoughts and feelings have surfaced continue to breathe and relax.

- Now intuitively tune in to the energy of the food you are holding. What is its vibration like? Does it have an energy field? Is it vibrant and life giving or inert? If this food had an energy color what would it be? If it could speak what would it be saying? Will it strengthen or weaken your body and your energy field?

- Know that you have a choice. This food's energy is probably not able to transform difficult and uncomfortable emotions or negative thoughts. If there is a positive feeling that you get from the food you are holding, absorb the good, positive energy without eating it. Ask yourself how to take care of yourself without eating the food you are holding.

Energy as Weight

We collect and absorb energy all day. From the friend who is having a difficult time to the coworker who sits close by and has a headache, we unconsciously absorb the emotional, mental, and physical issues and problems of those we care about and even those whom we barely know. We are energy and we are always connecting, merging, and reaching out to the energy world that surrounds us.

Have you ever talked to someone and become exhausted as they shared their account of recent problems and issues? After expressing their stress and anxiety, he or she may walk away feeling lighter while you heavily shuffle out the door. Some seek out others who they know they can give their worries and burdens to. Likewise, many loving, positive people take on the stress and pain of others, not realizing the negative impact that this will have on their emotional, mental, and physical health.

There is a very real connection between the energetic stress and burdens you absorb from others and your physical weight. Have you have ever had difficulty losing weight? No matter what you eat and how much you exercise, you are not able to lose those pounds and might even continue to gain? Do you suddenly seem to gain weight even when you eat the same amount of food day after day? If this sounds like you, the energy that you are absorbing from others may be to blame.

Your unconscious mind may be converting the excess energy you have absorbed into physical pounds. The unconscious mind does not evaluate and reason. It simply responds to the information and data at hand. If you are overburdened and heavy with energy, the body will simply manifest more physical weight.

By strengthening and clearing your energy field of the problems, stress, and aches and pains you have absorbed from others, you can protect yourself from accumulating unnecessary energetic weight. You can use the following meditation on a regular basis to release energetic baggage and lose weight.

MEDITATION: ENERGY CLEANSING AND CLEARING FOR WEIGHT LOSS

- Close your eyes and take a long deep breath, and send the energy of the breath to any part of your body that is sore or tense or tight. Exhale the tension and stress. Take another breath and a long, deep, relaxing exhale.

- As you breathe imagine a translucent rainbow of light and color. Visualize yourself bathed in this rich stream of love, vibration, and energy. Relax, and allow these colors and vibrations to surround you.

- Continue to breathe and draw your awareness to the top of your head. Imagine white light streaming into your body. Breathe in this white light energy and ask that it dissolve and release any negative or toxic energy that you have willingly and unwillingly absorbed from an external source. Ask that it be sent into the white light and purified.

- Become conscious of a spiral of energy surrounding your head. Breathe white light into this area. Imagine your third eye opening. (The third eye is the sixth chakra, which is explained in detail in chapter 11.) Deep purples and indigo may appear. Continue to breathe energy into this area, releasing any negativity, stress, and tension.

- Move your awareness to the throat area. Allow the light to dissolve and release whatever you no longer need. Allow the inner voice of truth to emerge. Listen and breathe. Release limiting or negative thoughts and judgments that you have taken on from others.

- Become aware of your heart. Imagine white light flowing into this area and rich waves of love opening within you. Allow any pain, wounds, or grief to surface. Breathe and release any feelings and emotions that are not serving your highest good. Know that all you need to do to let go of feelings and emotions is to feel them as they surface. Ask that any energy that you have absorbed from others be released and sent into the light.

- Become aware of your solar plexus, feel its strength and vibrancy. Allow white light energy to flow into your stomach. Feel the presence of power within you. Breathe and release any shame or guilt and any thoughts and beliefs that restrict your power. Feel your power as vibrant vital life force energy.

- Move your consciousness into the area below your belly button. Imagine white light flowing into this area. Breathe in white light energy and release and let go of any limiting judgments about your sexuality and your ability to thrive in a relationship and care for yourself. Clear this area with the breath of love.

- Become aware of the base of your spine. Breathe white light energy into this area and feel your connection with the earth. Feel the earth supporting and loving you. The earth has called you into physical being. It loves you and supports you. Feel your oneness with all that is.

- Allow white light cleansing energy to flow through your entire body. It is complete love and wisdom. It flows through you and dissolves and releases any energetic baggage that you no longer need. Allow white light energy to expand through you, relaxing and energizing you.

- White light energy now extends about twelve inches from your body. It forms an orb of translucent light completely surrounding you. Stress and negativity continue to be released and only what is in your highest good can enter.

- Repeat an affirmation, either speak it aloud or write it down. Do this often and your unconscious will act on these positive statements.

For instance:

I let go of unnecessary weight. I am nurtured
  by vibrant source energy. I am the perfect weight.

Intuitive Energy Imbalance

Developing your intuition and utilizing it in your daily life requires energy. When I teach intuition development my students are always surprised by how tired they are by the end of a class. Most of us understand how exhausting a long day at work and a strenuous physical activity can be. Intuitively tuning in to energy information also draws from our energy reserves. Using your intuition on a regular basis will build up your energy muscle. The energetic capacity of your aura or energy field will increase as you continually use your intuition and absorb source energy. This is somewhat similar to the way weight lifting increases the size and strength of your muscles. By practicing the exercises in this book you will eventually begin to increase your energy reserves through aligning your intuition with higher vibrational source energy. This is your power source.

As your confidence with communicating, interacting, and connecting to high vibration energy increases, it is important to integrate it into every aspect of your mind, body, and spirit. If you do not do this you may become energetically imbalanced. How does this happen?

Intuitive energy can be seductive. Communicating with and opening to higher vibrations of energy can be soothing, invigorating, calming, exciting, and reassuring. When we realize our inner power and catch a glimpse of our authentic and eternal spiritual self, we are never the same. The material world can suddenly be a bit boring and harsh. For some people the allure of working with higher vibrational energy is all-encompassing. They may want to leave their old lives behind. Their jobs and career now feel like a waste of time. There is no longer meaning in the mundane and they desire to quickly leave behind the old and venture deeper into the spirit realms. Some people may feel as if they can no longer relate to their family and friends and even their spouse or partner. When you increase the capacity of the higher vibrations of your aura you may experience these and other physical, mental, spiritual, and emotional side effects.

Common Signs of Higher Vibration Energy Imbalance

- Sensitivity to light and noise

- Headaches

- Insomnia

- Lightheadedness

- Lack of appetite

- Lack of interest in work, friends, hobbies, social situations

- Spaciness, disorientation

- Absorption in daydreaming and fantasy

- Being distracted by spontaneous psychic visions and communication

- Experiencing breakthrough past life episodes

- Extreme feelings of elation followed by deep sadness

EXERCISE: BALANCING TECHNIQUES FOR INTUITIVE AND HIGHER VIBRATION AND ENERGETIC IMBALANCE

If you are experiencing any of these kinds of feelings and experiences, it is important to recognize that you are in the midst of a profound transformation. Once your intuitive spiritual energy has been ignited and unified with the conscious ego self, a life-changing process is in progress. You can help this process go more smoothly by integrating and assimilating the higher vibrations of energy into your physical body.

In metaphysical thought, the term "grounding" is understood as the full integration of the spirit within the physical body. It is being awake and alert, connected to the here and now and at the same time fully present within one's spiritual essence and energy. Certain grounding techniques and practices will help your mind, body, and spirit to operate as one. Once your equilibrium is restored you will experience a renewed sense of connectedness to both the spiritual and physical realms.

These simple practices will help restore energetic equilibrium.

- Walk in nature

- Garden

- Lift weights

- Practice yoga

- Get a massage

- Sweat in a sauna or steam room

- Laugh and share a meal with friends

- Walk a dog

- Ride a horse

- Eat root vegetables

- Eat meat or fish

- Watch comedy

- Volunteer to help those in need

- Drink plenty of water

- Swim

- Take a hot bath with invigorating herbal scents

- Walk along a river or the seashore

- Be creative—paint, sing, or write poetry

- Go barefoot outdoors

- Avoid negative people and situations

- Sit by a campfire

- Do repairs to your home

- Go fishing

- Have a reflexology session

MEDITATION: GROUNDING BREATH

Close your eyes and take a long deep breath. Move the energy of the breath through the body and release any stress and tension through the exhale.

Breathe white light energy down through the top of the head. Send the energy of the breath through the body; imagine exhaling it through the solar plexus. Place one hand above the head and the other hand on your abdomen. Continue to breathe.

Take another breath down through the top of the head. Send this breath down to the soles of your feet. Exhale and repeat this breath a few times.

Now imagine breathing energy up through the soles of your feet. As you do this, imagine the energy of the earth moving up through the body. Place one hand on the abdomen and one hand above the head. Imagine that your hands form a white light container of energy that completely surrounds you. Exhale through the solar plexus. Repeat this breath.

Continue to breathe energy from the earth up through the soles of the feet. Move this energy up into the body and exhale through the top of the head. Repeat this breath.

Breathe down through the top of the head and up through the soles of the feet. Place both hands on your abdomen. Feel energy in the palms of your hands, send it through the body, and back to the abdomen. Continue this breath and exhale through the solar plexus. Repeat until you feel yourself centered and in the body.

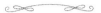

To be an effective medical intuitive it is essential to have good energy health. Not only will you be healthy, have more robust physical energy, and attract positivity into your life, your intuition will be more exacting and reliable. In the next section you will discover the unique way that you are already intuiting health information.

Section 2

Your Specialty: Discover
Your Medical Intuitive Type

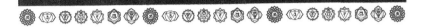

3

DISCOVER YOUR MEDICAL INTUITIVE TYPE

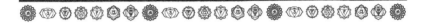

Your body, mind, and spirit are always communicating to you. You receive their messages through your innate intuition. Although you may not always be aware of it, you intuit health energy information through your thoughts, emotions, your physical body, or your energy field. I call these four different modalities of intuiting your medical intuitive type. Once you know how you to naturally intuit, it is easier to become aware of intuitive health messages and further develop this ability.

The following quiz will provide you with insight into your innate medical intuitive type. You are likely a combination of more than one type and some people are nearly equal with all of the four types.

QUIZ: MEDICAL INTUITIVE TYPE INDICATOR
Scoring
3 points=most of the time, 2 points=sometimes, 1 point=rarely

1. When in the company of someone who is ill or in pain, have you ever felt their aches and pains as if they were your own?

2. Have you ever known something about a health condition of another without knowing how you know it?

3. Do you feel others' feelings and have a sense of how they may be influencing their health?

4. Have you ever had a dream that provided you with insight into your health or someone else's?

5. Are you interested in giving and/or receiving hands-on healing?

6. Do you have an interest in the science behind mind, body, and spirit awareness and healing?

7. Do you feel the feelings of others who are miles and miles away when they are undergoing difficulties?

8. Can you sense or see the auras around people, animals, or plants?

9. When touching another have you ever received information about him or her and not known how you know it?

10. Does being in the company of negative people affect your health?

11. Do both positive and negative feelings and emotions affect your health?

12. Do you have an interest in energy medicine?

13. Have you ever picked up an antique piece of jewelry or held an object belonging to another and felt a distinctive vibration or energy coming from it?

14. Do you like exploring alternative and innovative healing techniques and tools?

15. Are you empathetic, caring, and have a desire to help others heal?

16. Can you feel others' energy as a buzzing or vibration?

17. Do you feel stronger, more connected, and full of energy when you are in the midst of positive people?

18. Do you know what others are thinking and how this may be affecting their health?

19. Have you ever experienced a physical healing after resolving a past emotional wound or difficulty?

20. Do you ever have a sense that there is an unseen spiritual presence close by?

21. Even when you are by yourself in nature, do you not feel alone?

22. Do you use positive thinking or affirmations to improve your health?

23. Do you believe that love can heal all?

24. Have you ever seen or felt a dull gray energy around someone who is ill?

25. Have you ever spontaneously intuited unknown facts about another's health just by looking at them?

26. Have you ever known what would heal or cure another's illness or disease and not known how you know it?

27. Have you ever had insight into the emotional root cause of another's illness?

28. Have you ever felt or seen a dull, dark shadow around another and knew that they were ill or about to become ill?

29. Do you use medicinal herbs when you are not feeling well, and do you have a sense of which ones will be most helpful?

30. Have you ever had a great idea for a revolutionary health system or invention?

31. Do you elicit the help and healing intervention of the angelic realm during times of difficulty and illness?

32. Do you feel that a loved one on the other side has ever alerted you to a health problem?

Scoring
3 points=most of the time, 2 points=sometimes, 1 point=rarely

	A		B		C		D
1		2	3		4		
5		6	7		8		
9		10	11		12		
13		14	15		16		
17		18	19		20		
21		22	23		24		
25		26	27		28		
29		30	31		32		
total							
	A		B		C		D

Add your totals for column A, B, C & D.

- If your highest sum is A you are a physical medical intuitive.

- If your highest sum is B you are a mental medical intuitive.

- If your highest sum is C you are an emotional medical intuitive.

- If your highest sum is D you are a spiritual medical intuitive.

- If your score totals are close or equal to more than one intuitive type, you exhibit the intuitive qualities of one, two, three, or even all four types. This is normal and will be quite helpful in developing your intuition.

Now that you are aware of your intuitive type, you are ready to learn more about what this means by exploring the unique intuitive characteristics and potential of each type. The following chapters will provide you with insight into all four medical intuitive types.

4

COMPASSIONATE INSIGHT: EMOTIONAL INTUITION

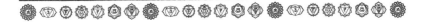

Emotional intuitives intuit energy information primarily through their emotions. Attuned to the vibrations of divine love and emotional energy, they experience a wide range of emotions and desire meaningful and heartfelt connections. Emotional intuitives naturally absorb others' feelings and emotions and the emotional energy of events near and far. Clairempathy, the ability to feel and perceive another's emotions as one's own, is a form of emotional intuition. Yet, while the focus of clairempathy is the ability to intuit the emotions, feelings, and sensations of others, emotional intuition also includes the ability to intuitively connect with the cosmic energy of divine love.

In the area of health and wellness, emotional intuitives' innate intuitive ability provides them with insight into the emotional wounds, pain, and the repressed emotions that affect their health and the health of others. They may be intuitively alerted to issues and problems with another's health through a sense of urgency or a sinking upset and persistent feeling. Often emotionally aware of illness before its onset, they may experience an undeniable impulse to reach out to a loved one weeks before he or she is ill. With kindness and caring they share their time and attention with those they intuitively feel need their help. Although this kind of attentive concern may seem unusual or surprising to the recipient, in time their emotional intuitive barometer is proven correct. Their clairempathic awareness soon becomes a source of comfort when a health crisis occurs.

Emotional Insight into Health

Emotional intuitives are on an intuitive journey to fully understand the link between illness and emotions. Have you ever been ill and intuitively knew that your poor health was connected to long-standing, deep, or repressed feelings of sadness, anger, frustration, or grief? Have you ever experienced relief from pain or healed an illness after forgiving another or letting go of a grievance? These are the kinds of experiences that inspire and help the emotional intuitive to become more aware of their powerful connection to emotional energy. Once an emotional intuitive understands how their emotions impact their health and well-being they tend to heal their past emotional wounds and focus on maintaining loving and positive emotions.

This is what happened with Kara. A thirty-six-year-old esthetician, she initially came to see me for advice in relationships. Attracted to immature men who initially shower her with attention, compliments, and a desire for constant contact, the fairy tale relationships always seemed to end with disappointment. Kara could not understand why she attracted men who came on strong but in time became controlling and possessive. Kara wanted me to tell her when she would meet her soul mate, a man who would love and respect her and not be threatened by her independent nature.

During my session with Kara, I expressed concerns about her current relationship. Like many emotional intuitives, she both enjoys emotional intensity and unknowingly gravitates toward being in relationships with those she feels she can help. Her current relationship was similar to many of her past ones. Even though the man she was seeing was attentive, the controlling behavior was already beginning. I told Kara that I did not intuitively see this ending well. She needed to become more comfortable with men who had better self-esteem. She was

picking men who were handsome but intense and emotionally immature. She wanted to heal their emotional wounds and help build their
confidence, but her efforts were only met with resistance.

The stress of her current relationship along with past heartaches
was affecting her self-esteem, robbing her of her power and lowering
her immune system. Eventually, I told her, this would not only lead
to more disappointment, it would also affect her health and make
her more prone to illness. Even though she was attracted to relationships that provided her with emotional intensity, the love she sought
seemed to elude her. The soul mate she desired would only come into
her life when she treated herself with love and compassion and expected the same from others.

I saw Kara about a year after our first reading. She came in for
another session and told me that she was recovering from a bladder
infection. Before this she had a bad case of the flu and before this she
had a developed a staph infection in what she thought was a minor
cut on her arm.

"In many ways I have had a difficult year," she told me. "I was sick
on and off for most of it and my boyfriend and I broke up and got back
together several times. I finally ended it about six weeks ago. One day I
was lying in bed, too sick to go to work, and it hit me. I was dozing off
and I could literally feel the toxic emotions of the relationship coursing
through my veins. It felt like poison. I intuitively knew that this was the
root of my recent illnesses. I now really understand that I need genuine
goodness and love in my life. I made a decision to spend my time with
kind and loving people who truly care for me. I am also listening to my
intuition more. It is really paying off. I am finally beginning to trust it."

Not only did Kara make a significant breakthrough in understanding how emotions were affecting her health, she was also able to break
the cycle of disappointing relationships. She began to forgive and love
herself and listen within to her intuition more. Eventually at a friend's
wedding, she met Brian. Although he did not initially stir up feelings
of passion and emotional intensity, she listened to her intuition and

accepted his dinner invitation. Six months later they are still going strong and she is happier and healthier than she has been in a long time.

Emotionally Intuiting Others' Health

Emotional intuitives often intuitively tune in to the emotional causes of others' illnesses, especially those people with whom they are close and care about. This comes so naturally to them that many emotional intuitives do not question their insights or feel that it is anything other than common sense.

For instance, when I did a reading for Sarah she asked me about her mother's health. I scanned her mother's body and was drawn toward her chest and lung area.

"I am feeling a problem with your mother's lungs. This feels chronic, likely since childhood," I told her. "It feels to me that your mother has trouble breathing, her lungs feel filled with mucous and inflamed. It feels like bronchitis."

Sarah listened and then confirmed my findings. "My mother had asthma as a child, now she has bronchitis or pneumonia at least once a year. Growing up, her parents were strict and emotionally absent. She was told she could speak only when she was spoken to and there were not a lot of fuzzy warm feelings in her home. I have always thought that this may have something to do with her health, and specifically her problems with her lungs. I have suggested she go to therapy and talk some of this out. I just think releasing these old memories and the pain connected to them would help her health improve."

Sarah's concern and intuitive observation of the energy behind her mother's health is fairly typical for an emotional intuitive. Because of their innate ability to intuit the emotional energy of others they will often tune in on the emotional influences that may be causing or contributing to disease or illness. Because others may not be aware of their own repressed emotions and how those emotions may be affecting their health, an astute emotional intuitive's insight can go unacknowledged and misunderstood.

Emotional Energy and Health

Emotions and health are indelibly linked. Eastern medicine has long been mindful of this connection. In many Eastern health systems, illness and imbalance in the physical body is associated with specific emotions. For example, in traditional Chinese medicine, problems with the spleen and stomach are related to worry, the liver and gall bladder to anger and frustration, the lungs and large intestine to sadness and grief, the kidney and bladder to fear and shock, and the heart and small intestine are affected by excess excitement.

Conventional Western medicine is becoming increasingly aware of the important role that emotions play in health and well-being. Physicians such as Andrew Weil, Deepak Chopra, and Christine Northrop have led the way in helping us to understand the connection between thoughts, emotions, beliefs, and our health. Medical intuitive researcher and physician Norm Shealy, MD, explores emotional and psychological issues to better understand and help cure and heal illness and disease.

Although everyone's physical health is affected by their emotions, an emotional intuitive is most prone to having an immediate physical reaction to emotional energy. It is not just their own emotions that affect them. The emotional energy that they unknowingly absorb from others and from the environment can have a significant impact on their health and well-being.

Because they are highly sensitized to emotional energy their tendency to absorb emotional vibrations can be either energizing or depleting. Positive emotions, such as joy, tranquility, and harmonious connections with others, increase emotional intuitives' daily available energy reserves and strengthen their physical body. Emotions such as fear, anger, grief, confusion, and unsatisfying and disruptive relationships deplete their physical energy, lower their immune system, and are often the root cause of illness.

Listen to Your Emotions

An emotional intuitive often intuitively tunes in to an illness or physical problem before it manifests. If you are an emotional intuitive, it is important to pay attention to puzzling and often subtle emotions such as nervousness, stress, and unease. Persistent unsettling emotions may be intuitive messages. At times these messages may be forewarnings of problematic issues with health and well-being. When you have these kinds of feelings and do not know why, take some time to listen within. Rarely do people regret paying attention to their intuited feelings. This is what happened to Gloria.

While driving her daughter to soccer practice one afternoon, Gloria, a mother of three, experienced a fleeting feeling of emptiness and grief. This made no sense to her. With a loving husband and family her days were full and active from morning to night. She quickly dismissed the feelings. But they did not go away. Several days later Gloria woke early in the morning with a hollow feeling in her chest and a lonely feeling in her heart. Again, she dismissed these feelings and got busy getting her children ready for school. Soon after, feelings of loneliness and emptiness became the norm. In response to these feelings, Gloria became as busy as possible. Surrounding herself with people, she thought, would drive the feelings of loneliness away. She became the president of the PTA at her children's school and signed up to teach Sunday school at her church. Still the feelings did not go away. The hollow feeling in her chest became heavier and was now accompanied by constant exhaustion. Then one afternoon on her way to pick up her children at school, she was struck with the unshakable feeling that something was not right. She knew that she was seriously ill. A shiver of fear ran up her spine and her palms became sweaty. She called her doctor as soon as she got home. A few days later her doctor ordered a series of tests, including a mammogram. A few weeks later Gloria had surgery to remove a tumor in her right breast. Several weeks of chemo followed.

Gloria did everything that her doctors recommended. Still, she knew that there was more to do to heal. She knew that she had to resolve the feelings of emptiness and grief that she intuitively felt were at the core of her illness.

This is when I met Gloria. She came to see me for help in understanding the connection between her health and the confusing emotions that preceded her illness. When I began the reading, her mother, who had passed over to the other side when Gloria was a young girl, was immediately present. As soon as I began to share her messages with Gloria she began to cry. A flood of emotion came pouring out. As I continued with the reading I discovered that Gloria's mother died in a car accident when Gloria was fifteen. This was the same age as one of Gloria's daughters. This had triggered the deep grief of loss that she had felt when her mother died. The oldest of three children and the only girl, Gloria had put aside her feelings of loss to care for her younger siblings. Now, despite her full life and loving family, those feelings were still present and in need of healing. Although Gloria had released much of the pent-up and repressed grief of losing her mother. She knew that to fully heal she had to do more. From a young age she had cared for and nurtured others and expected little in return. The empty hole in her chest of loneliness and sadness needed to be filled. She intuitively knew that she needed to take time for self-reflection. As difficult as it was to focus on her own needs, she knew that in order to heal she had to. Gloria began to extend the same compassion, nurturing, and care to herself that she did to others. Making time to meditate and pray on a daily basis, she opened herself to receiving divine love and compassion. She also made time in these sessions to intuitively feel the presence of her mother loving and caring for her from the spirit realm. Gloria fully recovered and was declared cancer free, and instead of constant heaviness in her chest she now feels a deep and abiding warm, loving presence.

The Healing Heart of the Emotional Intuitive

To develop medical intuition it is necessary for an emotional intuitive to harness the power and intelligence of emotional energy. Rightly used, emotional energy is a dynamic tool that can detect illness and uncover the origin and cause of an illness or disease and heal the body. To develop this ability, an emotional intuitive must first learn how to become aware of emotional energy and then paradoxically detach from it.

While emotional intuitives can feel emotions intensely, they cannot allow what they feel to define, control, and overly influence them. Instead of being tossed and turned in the tumultuous energy of emotions, emotional intuitives need to develop the ability to tune in to the quiet inner sanctuary of the heart. This is where the wise and loving intuitive voice of the spirit resides. Underneath the intensity of everyday feelings, peace and harmony radiate from the heart center. Emotional intuitives have an innate connection to the heart. This is where their true intuitive power resides. In the midst of strong, confusing, or intense emotions, know that you can focus your awareness within. Feel your feelings but do not become their slave. Once you connect with the quiet, loving intuitive self, emotions become its tool. You are then able to channel the power of the emotion of love and compassion to heal yourself and others.

Once emotional intuitives learn how to harness the power of emotional energy and heart centeredness, they can become sensitive and gifted medical intuitives. With an acute intuitive sensitivity to emotions, they can detect the toxic, repressed, and hidden emotional wounds of others. They innately know and understand the power that negative emotions have to influence and affect health. With a soulful drive and desire to heal, they encourage others to discharge and release unhealthy emotions and then replace them with healing rays of love and compassion.

Emotional Healing Modalities

To experience optimum health and well-being and to heal existing illness or disease, emotional intuitives tend to respond to emotive healing modalities. Because they intuitively absorb the emotions of others and the emotional energy of traumatic events, it is crucial that they practice some form of periodic emotional release. Since they tend to absorb emotional energy from external sources, they may not always be aware of the degree of their emotional toxicity. Unresolved, stifled, hidden, and unknown accumulated emotional energy is powerful.

The following emotive therapies can facilitate the release of emotional negativity and toxicity. A large number of emotional intuitives can be found participating in and assisting and healing others through these therapies.

Talk therapy that focuses on past and present emotional wounds and pain, especially therapies that promote detecting and letting go of repressed and emotional energy, revitalizes and heals the emotional intuitive. Powerful transformative healing for the emotional intuitive also comes through heart-centered meditation, opening to and receiving divine love, and forgiving self and others. Emotional intuitives have a special connection to the angelic realm. Intuitively connecting with angels through meditation and visualization or working with an intuitive practitioner who communicates with the angels can be beneficial for the emotional intuitive.

Expressive music, dance, and art therapy can facilitate the expression and release of emotional energy that is difficult to put into words. This can be especially helpful with negative emotional energy that has been absorbed from others. Emotional freedom technique (EFT) is a therapy that can quickly release and transform repressed and unhealthy emotional energy from the physical body. EFT is an intuitive system of tapping and applying pressure to specific meridian points in the body to release emotional energy blockages. A somewhat similar process is emotional polarity therapy that identifies toxic emotions in the body, releases them, and brings the body back into energetic balance and harmony.

Emotional intuitives love to help and serve. As medical intuitives they bring a special soothing sensitivity to tuning in to and healing the body, mind, and spirit.

Unlike emotional intuitives, mental intuitives intuit through thought and mind energy. In the next chapter you will learn how their natural ability to understand complexity serves them well as medical intuitives.

5

THE KNOWER:
MENTAL INTUITION

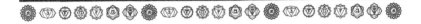

Mental intuitives absorb intuitive energy information through their thoughts. It is not unusual for them to intuitively receive fascinating truths and insights about various topics and subjects that they know little about. Their instantaneous intuitive knowing more often than not is proven to be correct. Mental intuitives tune in to the energy of the mind, the unconscious, and the collective consciousness. Their expansive intuitive thinking encourages them to be pattern and systems oriented. With the ability to see the big picture, mental intuitives strive for a cohesive, thorough understanding in their chosen areas of interest.

As medical intuitives, mental intuitives tend to be stimulated by challenges and can intuitively perceive the interconnectedness and interaction between the various systems of the body. They often receive health information through an internal instantaneous sense of knowing or through intuitive hearing. They can be excellent medical intuitive detectives, deciphering and uncovering the origins of illness and disease. When it comes to their own health, mental intuitives will often be alerted to physical issues through a simple and recurring sense of knowing or through a persistent inner voice.

Persistent Knowing

Clark was not my typical client. In his early sixties, he was a partially retired engineering consultant. A skeptic, he had little hope that I could help him. When he came into my office, he stated that he was referred to me by a friend of his wife. He told me that he wanted me to tell him anything I could about his health. By his demeanor and body language I knew he did not have high expectations that I could be of any help. I started to scan his body and was drawn toward his abdomen. I could see swollen red tissue and scarring.

"I can see a small scar in your abdomen," I told Clark. "The tissue is still swollen. Did you have an appendectomy?"

"I had surgery a couple of months ago for a ruptured appendix," he told me with a surprised look on his face. "Do you see anything else?"

I continued to scan his body, and for the most part he appeared to be healthy.

"I keep being drawn to the area where you had surgery. You seem to me to be in good health. I'm a bit concerned that you might have an infection in the surgical area."

Clark confirmed my perceptions. "I'm on an antibiotic. I've been back to my doctor and have also been to a couple of other ones. Something is not right. I just know it. Would you look harder and tell me what you see."

I once again focused on Clark's abdominal area. As I did this I reported my findings to Clark. "I feel thick tissue where the infection is. This tissue feels inert and without a life force. The more I look at this it feels like an object, like gauze or something." I hesitantly told him, "I think during surgery there may have been something left in you."

"Aha!" Clark loudly repeated a few times. "I knew it. As soon as I woke up after surgery, I knew something was not right. I don't know how I knew this, but this thought will not go away. Sometimes I hear an inner voice telling me to get this taken care of. It will not let me rest. I'm having constant pain in this area. Even with the antibiotics the pain and infection is not going away. I know that something was left in me during the surgery. You better believe that I'm not going to rest until I get this thoroughly checked out and taken care of."

Clark left my office a believer.

Health Thoughts of Others

Similar to their own health concerns, mental intuitives intuit information about others' health through their penetrating intuitive thought process, through an insistent sense of knowing, and through inner hearing. This most often happens with people the mental intuitive has a close relationship to, but it can happen with anyone, including strangers.

On her way to work on the train one morning, Suzi received a text message from a work colleague. Jen was ill and would not be coming in to work that day. When Suzi heard the news she had a moment of panic. Realizing that she would have to make a presentation on her own that day, her mind started racing as she mentally reviewed the bullet points and goals for the meeting. As she struggled to remember all of the important facts, her mind blanked for a moment. Pausing to look out of the window, she suddenly and instantaneously knew what was wrong with her colleague Jen. She quickly sent a text message to her.

"Do you have food poisoning?" she asked.

"I might. I thought it was a virus, though. The chicken I had last night at Kelly's Grill seemed a little off to me. How the heck did you know this?" Jen sent the message back to her.

"I have no idea. It just popped into my mind. Get better. I have today covered," Suzi replied.

It is often through these kinds of random thoughts and insights that a mental intuitive receives health energy information.

Absorbing Negative Thought

Negative thoughts, critical judgments of self and others, limited thinking, and pessimistic beliefs affect our health and well-being. The most powerful energy in the universe is love. It flows toward creative evolution, expansion, and growth. When our thoughts are positive and we flow in this current, our mind, body, and spirit are nurtured and we thrive. When our thoughts and beliefs are negative we block the flow of life-giving energy and our health suffers.

Likes attract likes. This universal law applies to energy. When we generate positive energy we intuitively attract more positive energy. When we generate negative thoughts we intuitively attract more negative energy. Unseen negative energy collects in thought form like clouds. When we unknowingly tap into these collective negative energy pools we perceive everything that we encounter through this perspective. The opposite of rose-colored glasses, our perception is gray and downcast. It can become difficult to break out of this spell. We may turn to antidepressants and addictive behavior and substances to self-medicate.

Mental intuitives live in thought energy, both the positive and the negative. Because of their innate tendency to unknowingly intuit the thought energy of others and collective thought they are especially prone to being affected and influenced by negativity.

Depression Through Generations

Patty came in for a medical intuition session. A retired school teacher, she loved to learn and was currently taking a few classes at the Duke Retirement Center. Like many mental intuitives she had a thirst for knowledge and collecting information.

When I intuitively tuned in to Patty I could feel an overall lack of energy.

"I feel that you are chronically exhausted," I told her. "Even your emotional energy feels depleted. I feel that you suffer from depression and I can feel a kind of tingling and tremors in your hands and feet. Have you also been losing weight?"

"Yes, but I don't mind losing weight," she answered. "It's the constant tiredness and feeling of depression that I don't understand. I have never been depressed and I have always had lots of energy. I don't know what's wrong with me."

I tuned in to Patty and an image of a woman appeared.

"I am not sure yet why this is important, but I see a woman who I feel is your mother. I get the impression that she worked hard all of her life. I feel that she passed over at about the age you are now. Is this true?"

"That's true. I am the age that my mother was when she died. She was a single mother for many years and worked all of her life. She died soon after retiring, never getting the time to relax and enjoy herself. Her mother died at about the same age. We work hard and then we die. Do you think that I'm going to die soon? I guess there is a part of me that believes that is my fate. My life has been similar to my mother's life in many ways. Since I retired from teaching I guess I've become a bit obsessed with this thought."

As Patty talked I saw a gray shadow overtake her. I realized that her belief that she would soon pass over was drawing the life force out of her.

"Can you imagine a different future for yourself?" I asked her. "Your life here is not done. There is still much for you to do and experience. But to have the energy to go forward you have to believe that this is possible. You are not your mother or grandmother. They both suffered with depression and died at about your age. You are creating this same scenario for yourself through your thoughts and by taking on their depressive energy. But this is not your fate, only if you want it to be."

Patty sat still for a moment then told me. "Thank you, I feel that a weight has been taken from me. I am going to commit to paying attention to my thoughts and thinking more positively."

On her way out the door, I stopped her. "Patty, take some B vitamins, especially B12. You need it."

"It's so funny that you're telling me this. The thought keeps coming to me that I need to take B12 vitamins," she told me. "I'm not even sure where this thought comes from. But it's good to know my intuition is on track."

Developing Medical Intuition

To develop medical intuitive expertise a mental intuitive must be able to differentiate ego-mind chatter from the wise intuitive inner voice. Because of their tendency to be intuitive magnets for random thought energy, mental intuitives may ignore and disregard important messages. Many of the intuitive health insights that we commonly receive may be subtle and understated. They often urge us to do things like eat more nutritious foods, exercise regularly, forgive another, release past hurt and anger, think positively, and get a health checkup. Unfortunately, we often choose to ignore these kinds of important but subtle messages. We can be lazy when it comes to making changes, and these suggestions may require disciplined effort.

Developing medical intuition requires an openness of mind, heart, and spirit. We have to be willing to receive information that we may not want to hear. Intuition speaks the truth. Our ego-based thoughts often tell us what we want to hear, or the thoughts do the opposite and scare us with fears and doubts. Intuitive messages might not always compliment us or make much sense. They usually surface as a persistent and quiet inner knowing or thoughts that come to mind over and over. In quiet moments, while driving the car, mowing the lawn, exercising, or upon waking in the morning or going to bed at night, be especially attentive to any insistent thoughts or messages.

Because of the constant stream of mental energy that moves through the mental intuitive's mind, a regular meditation practice is beneficial. Meditation provides us with the opportunity to discern the intuitive voice from mind chatter. Sitting in a calm place, closing the eyes, and listening within is a simple, beneficial, and invaluable practice. The still and silent intuitive voice can be better recognized and acknowledged.

A mental intuitive's most soulful desire is to bond with wisdom and truth. Once awakened to their intuitive gifts, they can evolve from intuitively absorbing and tuning in to the thought energy of others to connecting with the energy of divine mind. Because of their innate ability to intuit the lofty vibrations of universal truth, they inherently understand the power of consciousness.

The Power of the Mind

Mental intuitives can be found in many medical and therapeutic settings. Attracted by the lure of uncovering the unknown, medical intuitives are often medical and scientific researchers. Although it may seem counter to intuitive awareness, many scientists and innovative medical device and systems developers are driven by their intuition. Mental intuitives tend to be devoted and hard working. Once their intuition and curiosity is activated they do not easily walk away from a problem they believe they can solve.

Mental intuitives are also attracted to the potential of using the power of the mind to heal in a more direct way. Our awareness that the mind embodies the power to heal and create abundance and well-being goes back to the beginning of time. Most ancient healing practices, such as traditional Chinese and Ayurvedic medicine and indigenous medicinal traditions throughout the Americas, emphasize the link between the mind and the body. The belief that the diseased or ill physical body needed to be viewed as separate from the mind, emotions, and the spirit in order for healing to take place began in the modern Western world. However, despite the emphasis on isolating the physical body from nonphysical influences, there have been many pioneers in the Western world who understood and emphasized the mind-body connection. Ernest Holmes was one of them. In 1927 he established the Science of Mind, a philosophical and metaphysical movement. The core concept within this system is the understanding of God as infinite intelligence. Holmes believed that every individual has access to the divine mind from which all physical, mental, emotional, and spiritual healing flows. Science of Mind, New Thought, and Religious Science churches and similar spiritual and metaphysical practices appeal to many mental intuitives who innately understand the power within the individual to access divine mind for healing illness and disease.

Our thoughts are powerful. Edgar Cayce, probably the most prolific and successful medical intuitive, often spoke about the power of the mind. His most fundamental teachings encourage us to understand how, rightly used, the mind can heal and perform miracles and how, incorrectly used, it can create havoc and suffering. To heal and create well-being in every facet of their lives and the lives of others, mental intuitives can utilize their natural connection to divine mind.

Some of the most effective healing and wellness therapies for mental intuitives invoke and harness mind energy. Among one of the most widely known and practiced is hypnosis. Merriam-Webster Dictionary defines hypnosis as: *a condition that can be artificially induced in people, in which they can respond to questions and are very susceptible to suggestion.*

Hypnotherapy is the use of hypnosis for therapeutic purposes. Hypnotherapy can tap into the unconscious and uncover repressed or forgotten information that may be affecting health and well-being. The inner mind holds a perfect record of everything that we have ever thought, experienced, felt, said, and done. It also is the doorway through which universal wisdom and the healing power can be accessed. Once negative or dysfunctional information is discovered through hypnosis, it can be released and suggestions for healing introduced. Without resistance and interference from the conscious ego self, these positive suggestions are accepted by the inner mind and acted upon. Through hypnotherapy an individual can also access the collective consciousness and the divine mind. In this state of awareness many people have been able to gain important information about their health and illicit divine help and healing intervention.

There are at present many therapies and practices that use the power of the mind to transform and improve health and well-being. Among them is Neuro Linguistic Programming or NLP. Created by Richard Bandler and John Grinder in California in the 1970s, it is a system of re-programming mental thought patterns through language and nonverbal cues. Advocates of NLP have shown success in addressing problems such as phobias, learning disabilities, and some illnesses, as well as using NLP in conjunction with psychotherapy.

Affirmations are another mind-centered tool for healing that appeals to many mental intuitives. Affirmations are positive statements that address specific unconscious negative or detrimental beliefs. They replace limited patterns of thinking with higher truth. When you consistently feed the mind positivity, it manifests. Chronic negative thought patterns and beliefs manifest as illness, pain, and disease. Because mental intuitives intuitively absorb so much mental energy information, it is especially important for them to use affirmations to keep positive energy flowing into their consciousness.

A helpful affirmation for mental medical intuitives is:

My mind perfectly intuits all I need
  to know for healing myself and others.

Stimulated and energized by the complexity and interconnectedness of the mind, body, and spirit, mental intuitives usually enjoy the challenge of developing medical intuition. Although naturally gifted in their ability to tune in to the physical body, physical intuitives are more stimulated by the sensory depth they experience when intuitively connecting with others. They are the focus of the next chapter.

6

THE SENSOR:
PHYSICAL INTUITION

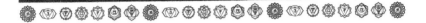

Physical intuitives have an innate intuitive connection to the physical world. With their unique intuitive relationship to nature and all living beings, they perceive the spirit within all of life. For the physical intuitive the material and physical is more than biology, it is the temple of the spirit. Practical and down-to-earth, their intuition is simple and direct and is usually experienced as a gut feeling or sensory stimulation. They also intuit through their hands and especially like to touch, hug, and hold hands with those they love.

Physical intuitives often unknowingly absorb energy information into the physical body. They may unsuspectingly soak in the illness, aches, and pains of others and feel them as their own. As medical intuitives they have the ability to identify illness, imbalance, and physical problems through observing the physical body and detecting signs that others cannot perceive. They can intuitively tune in to not-yet-manifested problems and issues through subtle physical and sensory impressions. Because their body is uniquely wired to receive and absorb energy information, even slight physical sensations can reveal a wealth of intuitive information.

This is what happened to Lucy, who fortunately listened to the subtle bodily sensations she was experiencing. When Lucy came in for a session, she was very enthusiastic. Although she had never had an intuitive reading, she told me that she was a true believer.

"A few years ago, I would have thought that all of this was nonsense," she told me. "I never gave intuitive and psychic abilities much attention. Then I had this experience. I'd like to tell you about it."

I told her that I'd love to hear it.

"Well I had this little twinge below my belly button. It really wasn't a pain or even a discomfort, but it was persistent and I felt uneasy about it. I went to my gynecologist and she did a complete exam. Everything looked fine. So I went to my regular doctor and he also did some tests. He told me the same thing. Everything seemed fine. I should have felt relief. But the strange thing was, I didn't. I still felt that something was not right. That little twinge would not go away. I waited several months and went back to the doctor. I think they thought that I was hysterical. Still, he found no issues. I went back another time a month or so after this. This time I went to a different doctor. They did the same tests, but this time they found something, a small tumor in my uterus. I had it removed a few weeks later. Because it was found so early, I'm now cancer-free. But what I want to know is how did I know that I had a problem months before it showed up?"

Intuiting Through the Senses

Physical intuitives are the most likely of all the intuitive types to ignore their intuitive abilities. They tend to live in the world of the five senses. What they cannot see, touch, taste, smell, and hear does not exist or is not tangible enough to believe in. They are "what you see is what you get" kind of people. Yet, the intuitive potential of the physical intuitive is just as vast and profound as the other types.

Although our five senses give us information about the physical and material world, physical intuitives can also intuit nonphysical energy information through their sense of touch, sight, hearing, and at times, even their sense of smell. Within their physical senses is the refined sensitivity to access intuitive energy information. What they hear, taste, smell, see, and touch transports them beyond the physical and into pure essence. This happens quite naturally. For instance, physical intuitives can look at someone and receive energy health information or hold someone's hand and know if they are about to get ill.

Maria is the mother of three children. Like many parents she is able to look at her children and know if they are coming down with a bug or virus before a fever or other telltale signs emerge. It was only when she began to look at others and spontaneously know the state of their health that she and others began to take notice.

One Saturday her oldest daughter's best friend Annie spent the afternoon playing at Maria's home. When Annie's father Arthur came to pick her up, Maria answered the door. Welcoming him into her home, she took one look at him and knew that something was not right.

"Have you ever had your tonsils out?" she abruptly asked him.

Startled by this unexpected question, he hesitated for a moment, then said. "No, why do you ask?"

Surprised by her own question, Maria simply laughed and said, "Oh, just humor me. I have been with my kids all week."

Maria went to get his daughter and they were soon on their way.

Several weeks later, Maria received a phone call from Arthur's wife. "Can Annie play with your daughter this Saturday?" she asked. "Arthur is having his tonsils out on Friday."

"Sure," Maria said. "I would love to have Annie here this weekend."

"Thank you, I owe you one," Arthur's wife replied. "By the way, Arthur told me that a few weeks ago you asked him if he'd had his tonsils out. How did you possibly know something was wrong? This came on so suddenly. We didn't know that they needed to come out until a week ago. How could you have known?"

"He just looked to me to be a bit pale and his voice seemed congested to me," Maria tried to explain. "I remember the same symptoms before my son Jeffery had his tonsils out. Arthur just seemed to have the same look that he did."

"That is a bit remarkable. Don't you think?" Arthur's wife responded.

"Not really," said Maria. "It happens all the time to me. I can take one look at someone and know the state of his or her health. I can feel it in my own body. Give him my best."

Talk to Your Body

For the physical intuitive the key to developing medical intuition lies in becoming conscious of their innate intuitive ability to perceive nonphysical energy. Emotional, mental, and spiritual intuitives are more comfortable with energy and essence. For the physical intuitive the idea of intuitively communicating with energy may be too abstract and elusive. Yet, once they understand that their natural inclination to discern and tune in to the physical body through their senses is a form of intuitive and psychic ability, physical intuitives may intuit health information with more natural ease than the other types.

One of the most effective ways for physical intuitives to discover their innate receptiveness to absorbing the energy of others is through a practice called body talk. Although this is useful for the physical intuitive, all intuitive types can benefit.

Try this: Become aware and focus on any areas of pain, tension, or tightness in your body. Once an area is located, tune in to this area and imagine that the energy you are connecting with is a color. Begin to communicate with this color. You might want to ask if this energy is yours or someone else's. Expect a response. Most of the time, you will quickly be able to discern if this energy is your own or if you have absorbed if from a source outside yourself. If this energy has been absorbed into your body from another, make the intent to release it. If this energy is yours, continue to dialogue with it to better understand and heal it.

Body talk is a skill that is similar to one that you will practice and use in medical intuitive body scans. It is valuable for all types, but may be especially helpful for the physical intuitive to become more conscious of the energy information they are absorbing.

How Healers Absorb Energy

Physical intuitive healers who practice hands-on techniques like chiropractic or massage therapy are especially prone to absorbing the energy information of others into their body.

Mariah is a popular acupuncturist and yoga teacher. When she came to see me for a session she was frustrated and confused.

"I am continuously exhausted. For years I have studied nutrition and Chinese medicine. I know the right things to do to be healthy. Yet, I cannot understand what's wrong with me. Some days I just want to sit and do nothing. I cancel appointments because I am just too tired to go to work," she told me.

When I looked at Mariah's physical and subtle energy, I saw and felt the energetic heaviness that she spoke of. Her body seemed to have large, concentrated areas of stagnant energy. Her energy field was dull and also felt heavy. Life force energy is luminous and in constant motion. Mariah's energy was the opposite. I intuitively knew that she was absorbing the energy of others. Once absorbed within our own system we cannot heal another's energy. It only weighs us down and can cause us physical, mental, emotional, and spiritual problems.

"Mariah, tell me how you work with your acupuncture clients. Do you use your intuition to gain further understanding of their physical ailments?" I asked her.

"Yes, I use my intuition all the time. Once they are lying on my table I scan their body before I place the needles. Then I tune in to my body. I know where their energy blocks are because I can feel my client's energy through my own body," Mariah explained.

"You're a physical intuitive," I told her. "When you tune in to your body to discover the blocks in your patients you are absorbing their energy. The problem is that while you are able to remove their blockages through acupuncture, their energy blocks are still within you. This is what's making you tired and exhausted. There is another way to do this without absorbing your client's energy. Let me explain it to you."

Learning to Trust Energy

To develop medical intuition a physical intuitive must become aware and trust the existence and wisdom of energy. Because they intuit through the body, physical intuitives often depend on what is physical to open the door to the unseen. When they touch another they may feel the soft hum of inner vibration. When holding an object, an advanced physical intuitive can feel the subtle stirring of energy that it emits. Standing in the forest, walking along on a beach, or simply looking out the window into a garden, they can naturally tune in to and blend with the vibrational frequency.

Developing the ability to perceive energy outside of the body's physical form is their challenge. Although medical intuition involves tuning in to the physical body, it is not necessary that the physical body is present. Energy, spirit, and intuition exist outside of time and space. Although the body appears to be a solid mass, it is actually energy vibrating at a low and dense frequency. Once a physical intuitive becomes aware of this they can better tune in to the subtle frequencies beyond physical matter. Instead of absorbing energy into their body they can sensitize their intuitive senses to tune in to and receive energy information before they absorb it.

Professions with Touch

Both conventional and alternative health care systems are populated with physical intuitives. With the ability to tune in to the physical body, the organs, and other systems, they can be natural diagnosticians. They are attracted to careers in medicine that give them the opportunity to work with the tangible and physical. Health fields such as orthopedics, sports medicine, osteopathy, chiropractic, surgery, and dental are populated with physical intuitives. They are also attracted to massage and physical therapy. There is a certain ease and confidence that these intuitives have when dealing with the physical health of others.

The physical intuitive's body is a vibrational transmitter of energy. This makes them especially suited to give and receive healing energy through touch. They are often attracted to professions where they are able to participate in connecting with others in this way. Many physicians, surgeons, and massage therapists transmit healing energy to their patients through physical touch. Working with others activates and stimulates their intuition. Having a physical inuitive as a doctor, body worker, or physical therapist also often comes with the extra bonus of receiving healing energy.

The Body as a Doorway to Spirit

For the physical intuitive the body is the doorway to spirit. They are revitalized and energetically uplifted when they tap into its inner wisdom. As medical intuitives, physical intuitives have an intimate connection with the physical body. It is their spiritual home. Some intuitive skills like clairvoyance, which is the ability to see energy information, may not come as naturally to them as to the other types. But their intuitively sensitive senses make up for it. They simply perceive more and deeper than others. Their sense of touch is especially intuitively penetrating. Psychometry, which is the ability to hold an object or look at a photo and receive energy information from it, comes naturally to them. Physical medical intuitives are able to intuitively tune in to others' health in this same way. Simply holding another's hand or looking at a photo can reveal insightful energy health information. Understanding the wisdom of the body and activating the healing potential within all living things is their special magic.

Physical intuitives are usually kinesthetic people who need to move, commune with nature, and participate in activities that stimulate the connection between their body and spirit. You will find physical intuitives scaling mountains, kayaking down rivers, and walking quietly in the woods. Not only do they love nature, they are able to activate the divine healing energy within it. They have an affinity and special bond with crystals and herbal and plant spirit medicine, flower essences, and essential oils.

They are drawn to and naturally understand Native American and other indigenous healing practices. Any traditions that elicit the wisdom and power of nature and animal spirits may get their attention. Physical intuitives are also attracted to spiritual and physical-oriented activities like yoga, quo jung, and martial arts.

I have a client, Tammy, whose life changed when she took a class in kung fu. A forty-five-year-old state employee and mother of three children, she had been searching for a spiritual path for years. One evening on her way home from work she saw a banner advertising a kung fu class. That night she dreamed that she was skillfully flying through the air as a martial arts expert. Dancing and leaping in moves that she intuitively knew how to execute, she felt more alive than she had in a long time. The next day, Tammy signed up for beginners kung fu class and she has never looked back. Although Tammy had never participated in anything like this before, she was a natural. After her initial beginners class she started to take a class one or two nights a week. Soon she was exploring the spirituality of kung fu and realized that her spirit came alive when she was engaged with a physical practice. Over the course of two years, Tammy lost thirty pounds and became a toned athlete, disciplined in mind and spirit.

"I have been searching for so long for a spiritual connection," she told me. "I have taken workshops and read books about angelic communication, spirit guides, past lives, and energy healing. But I have never felt so in touch with my spirit as I do when I practice kung fu."

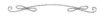

As medical intuitives, physical intuitives have a natural thirst and drive to tune in to the physical body. Almost at the opposite end of the spectrum, spiritual intuitives are equally attuned to the subtle energy body. In the next chapter you will learn more about the intuitive talents of the spiritual intuitive.

THE ENERGY ARTIST: SPIRITUAL INTUITION

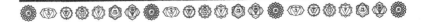

O f all of the intuitive types, spiritual intuitives are the most comfortable with essence and energy. They have a visceral connection to energy and the spirit world that may confound the other types. Unlike physical intuitives they do not need the physical form to perceive energy. Mental intuitives intuit though their thoughts, and emotional intuitives intuit through their emotions. For the spiritual intuitive energy information is received in a less tangible way, through their energy field.

The aura or energy field is a subtle luminous halolike field of energy that surrounds every living thing. Spiritual intuitives are intuitively sensitive to the higher vibrations of the energy field. Some spiritual intuitives are able to perceive it through intuitive clairvoyant sight as a faint glow of luminous energy surrounding people, plants, and animals. More advanced spiritual intuitives can tune in to the energy field and receive the important energy information contained within it.

Spiritual intuitives approach medical intuition a little differently than the other types. Physical, mental, and emotional intuitives innately tune in to the physical body and understand how emotions, thoughts, diet, exercise, and lifestyle affect health. A spiritual intuitive may instead perceive the physical body as a vehicle for the spirit. They tend to prefer to focus on energy as opposed to physicality and may intuit influences that the other types fail to perceive. Abstract factors such as past lives, energy attachments, and life purpose are more likely to get their attention. For the other types, these influences may seem more obscure and less important.

A Warning in a Dream

Spiritual intuitives usually have a rich dream life. In their dreams they may visit otherworldly realms, and converse with spirit beings and angels. They may also have intuitive dreams that provide them with present, past, and future insight and information about their family and friends. It is not unusual for a spiritual intuitive to be alerted through a dream about a health condition or illness. At times they might also dream of another's health and receive specific remedies for healing.

Tatiana, a college student, came to see me to help her understand a surprising dream that foretold a potential health problem. When she came into my office she sat down on my couch and immediately started talking.

"I had a hard time falling asleep one night," she told me. "I usually have no problems in this area. After lying awake for what seemed forever. I finally dozed off, only to be startled awake by a dream. In it I was in the woods, next to a river, and even though it was a sunny day, I had an ominous feeling. That was my first dream."

Tatiana continued, talking a little faster now. "The funny thing is the following weekend I had plans to go kayaking with some friends. When I got to the river, I was a little nervous. It looked so much like the dream scene. But it turned out to be a great day. Everything went fine, no accidents or problems of any kind. Then a few days later I had another dream. In it I was looking at my back in the mirror. I had a feeling of urgency, but I could not understand why. The next morning I kept thinking about the dream so I looked at my back in the mirror. To my surprise, I saw a big red mark but I couldn't make out what it was. I had my roommate take a look and she found a big tick in the middle of my back. I went to the school nurse and she put me on antibiotics. I am still trying to understand if this dream was warning me of the tick bite."

Tatiana's dream was a precognitive warning of a health condition. Through the dream images and the feelings she had in the dream, she knew to pay attention to it. The meaning and messages that our dreams contain are not always obvious. Dreams often speak to us through symbols, metaphors, and peculiar characters. If you do not fully understand a dream's message, pay attention to the feelings you experienced in it or in the morning when you wake. Ask for another dream or intuitive message that will help you to further understand what it is trying to tell you.

Perceiving Energy

Spiritual intuitives often receive energy information through inner or outer intuitive sight. This ability can surface through the appearance of dreamlike images and visions. Because they are sensitized to the energy field or aura, they may also perceive the presence of others' auras. For some, the sudden emergence of visions, luminous light, and streams of color around another can be surprising and confusing. At times this may also be perceived as a shimmering glow being emitted from a beloved pet, or a soft purple shade of color surrounding a tree or flowers. This psychic phenomenon may abruptly materialize as a result of reading and learning more about intuition and the paranormal. It may also occur during times of extreme stress, heightened joy, or periods of grief. There may also be no obvious cause or reason behind the sudden ability to see energy, images, and visions.

This is what happened to Eric. His ability to perceive energy happened one day at work. An MRI technician, he has worked in a conventional medical setting for many years. Drawn to help others, his job gives him the opportunity to work one-on-one with others who are often confused and searching for answers to their health problems. He contacted me in hope of understanding what he was experiencing and how to further develop what he believed was the sudden emergence of psychic ability.

I gave Eric a reading over the phone. Before I could begin the session, he told me, "I thought that I had seen everything. One day while reading Joe's chart, my patient who was due to arrive any minute, I glanced up at the door just as he walked in. To my surprise I saw a dull film-like color around his head. Joe was coming in that day for a brain scan. Suffering with increasingly painful migraine headaches for several months, his doctor thought an MRI was in order. When I saw this gray color surrounding him, my heart sunk. I knew the MRI would reveal a brain tumor. I am not sure how I knew. This had never happened before. A short time later his doctor told him the difficult news. Since then, this same thing happens every once in awhile. I never know when, but I have gotten pretty good at knowing what certain colors mean. Today I saw a bright, shining gold color around a little girl. I was relieved. I knew that there was nothing seriously wrong with her health and that she would recover."

Spiritual intuitives often have a sense of the energy surrounding others without seeing it in a visual three-dimensional way. Sometimes they perceive it through inner sight. Much of the time when this spontaneously happens people feel as if they are making it up with their overactive imagination.

When I was working as an art therapist for young people, I found that many of the young people I worked with associated certain colors with certain people. It was so common that I developed an exercise to help the kids better tune in to this skill. In this exercise I would ask the students to draw themselves and others in colors that indicated their feelings, mood, and thoughts. They took to this naturally and it became a useful tool for them to identify and express their feelings and thoughts. At times they would describe and share more about one of their parents or another student by telling me that he or she was dark blue or red or some other shade or color variation. They rarely visually saw these colors surrounding themselves and others in a three-dimensional way. Instead their inner sight helped them to perceive it more through their imagination.

Intuiting Health Energy

For the spiritual intuitive, who tends to enjoy hanging out in pure spiritual energy, reality can be lofty and equally as elusive as their intuitive awareness. Their challenges in developing medical intuition are in some ways nearly opposite of the physical intuitive. While the physical intuitive needs to develop sensitivity to essence and energy, the spiritual intuitive must focus on the physical.

Spiritual intuitives are not always interested in physical reality. Of course they have to live in it and care for the body as much as anyone. Yet these functions are not necessarily where their passions lie. They would much rather be conversing with the angels or experiencing the cosmic flow of energy. However, when they focus their natural gifts on the physical they can make a significant impact in the health and well-being arena. Their innate awareness of energy dynamics and the tendency to visually perceive energy allows them a unique view of the physical body.

Spiritual intuitives have a natural connection to the spirit world. They are more likely than the other types to receive messages and communicate with the other side. Emotional intuitives feel the soothing vibrations of divine love. Physical intuitives often intuitively converse with plants, power animals, and stones and crystals, while mental intuitives intuitively tap into the collective higher mind. The spiritual intuitive is the most versed in accessing energy information from the spirit realm. This might be through loved ones on the other side, spirit guides and teachers, angels, archangels, or divine-source energy.

A Loved One Shares a Health Message

Quite often our loved ones who have passed over are aware of our health issues before we are and try their best to send us messages.

Jessica was excited to begin her session with me. A kindergarten teacher in her early thirties, she told me that this was her first reading.

I began the reading and quickly became aware of Jessica's desire to have a child. She and her husband had been trying for almost a year and she was becoming concerned. After explaining how her diet—which was heavy in sugar, dairy products, and carbohydrates—was slowing down the conception process, I asked her if she had any other questions.

"I'm always concerned about my parents," she said. "Is there anything that I need to know about my mother?"

As Jessica was asking me about her mother, I could feel the presence of someone from the spirit world come close.

I told her, "I know that you want me to take a look at your mother. But, a woman in spirit, who I feel is your grandmother, keeps trying to get my attention. She is telling me that she is concerned about your mother's health and she has been trying to get a message to her…and to you."

"That's funny that you're saying this. I was dozing off while reading a book one afternoon and I saw an image of my grandmother's face. She seemed concerned, but I didn't know why. I told my mother about it and she said that she had felt her too. But we don't know why."

"Yes, your grandmother is anxious to get a message to you," I told her. "She shows me an image of your mother. I get the impression from your grandmother that your mother has been tired lately. Your grandmother tells me that diabetes is in the family. She wants your mother to get her blood sugar checked. Your mother needs to change her diet and it would also help if she lost a little weight."

"My grandmother had diabetes later in life," Jessica explained. "She didn't take very good care of herself. She died in her early sixties, much too young. We all really miss her. Can you ask her if she knows anything about me having a baby? She seems to know a lot about my mother's health."

As soon a Jessica asked the question, her grandmother began to answer.

"Your grandmother is holding a baby. She wants to have some time with her before she comes into the physical world. She sends you a similar message to the one I began with. Avoid eating too much dairy and sugar, it's creating heavy mucus. Your grandmother says not to worry.

Your baby is just about ready to make her debut. She just wants a little more time with her."

Energy Healing

Many spiritual intuitives gravitate toward interests, hobbies, and careers that involve energy awareness, spirituality, and esoteric and mystical topics. In the area of health and wellness, energy medicine has a particular allure for the spiritual intuitive. Energy medicine, also called energy healing, spiritual healing, or energy therapy, is the practice of channeling healing life force energy to yourself or another individual, group, or animal for the purpose of healing and improving health. There are a few different ways to transfer healing energy to others. Hands-on prayer or faith healing and distance healing, where the practitioner and client are not in the same physical location, are the most common.

Energy healing has been practiced for centuries. The belief that a higher form of energy can move through an individual and heal likely dates back to the beginning of time. Hippocrates believed that the power of nature moving through an individual had the power to cure illness and disease. In the Bible, Jesus lays his hands on the sick and lame and they are instantly healed.

Today energy medicine is becoming more widely accepted as a complementary and alternative medicine. Most practitioners learn specific techniques for accessing and applying healing energy to self and others. Reiki is a Japanese healing technique that can be either practiced by the laying on of hands or through distance healing. It is based on the belief that life force energy can be transmitted through an individual to another for physical, mental, emotional, and spiritual healing. Quantum Touch, a similar life force energy healing modality, is a therapy that incorporates physical touch, breath work, and body awareness meditations.

Many spiritual intuitives practice meditation and have rich inner lives. They may pray to God, the goddess, nature, angels, and universal life force energy for healing for self and others. With little need for worldly recognition, some spiritual intuitives prefer to work in secret, sending healing to others and to the planet. Monks, nuns, hermits, and even the modern-day quiet office worker who is rarely noticed may be broadcasting silent rays of healing energy far and wide.

Jada is a busy mom of three kids, all of whom are in elementary school. A couple of mornings and afternoons a week she picks up a vanload of kids as part of her carpooling responsibilities. I met Jada many years ago before she had children. During our work together I got to know her as a kind and compassionate healer. Being a spiritual intuitive, she loved communicating and connecting with the spirit realm and learned and practiced energy healing. She was thrilled when she learned that she was pregnant, but also a little apprehensive.

"I am so excited to become a mother," she told me. "But I'm also a bit nervous. How will I be able to spend time meditating and pursuing my spiritual interests? I don't know how this will all work out. But I want to be a good mom and I will do whatever it takes."

I did my best to assure her that she would be a great mom and still be connected with her spiritual interests.

I did not see too much of Jada once her first child was born. She did manage to come in for a session in between the births of her second and third children and she seemed to be adjusting just fine. Although she was very busy, her ability to juggle all that needed to be done and incorporate time for her spiritual interests was impressive. It was several years after the birth of her third child that we met again. She came in for a reading and to better understand her recent healing adventures.

When I began the session with Jada, I was impressed with her energy field. The translucent waves of turquoise, magenta, and golden light that I saw in her energy field told me she was surrounded by angels and powerful healing energy. As I tuned in to the luminous energy that seemed to cascade all around her, I knew that she was being used as a channel of healing for others, especially children. As I explained this to her she excitedly began to tell me more about her recent healing activities.

"I'm part of a school carpool. I pick up six kids and bring them to and from school several days a week. One morning last year I was driving with the kids and I looked in my rearview mirror and saw a luminous glow of gold and white energy surrounding them. I could see the health and vitality that they were emitting. Over time these luminous lights became more defined. Eventually I could see each child's energy field and discern more about them through the color and energy that they emitted. One day after picking up the kids I noticed that one young girl no longer had her normal luminous shine. The next day I learned that she was sick with a high fever and was out of school for over a week. Soon after this I noticed a similar low-emitting energy in another child. But this time I decided to see if I could help. I breathed deeply and imagined myself connecting to a higher vibrational energy. I saw this as white light and I sent this to the young boy until I felt the energy completely surround him. I continued to send him healing energy. Eventually I could see the boy's energy brighten up. I saw him a few days later and he seemed fine. I later heard that his family had all come down with a bad virus, but he had escaped any illness. I continued to do this whenever I felt that a child needed healing. Then one day as I was driving I saw an image of a woman in my mind's eye. I didn't know who she was, but she seemed tired and ill and she looked at me with sad eyes. I wasn't sure what to do. So I did the same thing that I had been doing with the kids. I sent her healing energy and kept doing this until her energy field seemed to brighten up and become stronger. This happens every once in a while; I may be driving, cooking dinner, playing with the kids, or meditating, and I see a vision of someone in my mind's eye who asks for healing. Sometimes I know the person. Maybe it's a family member or friend, but most of the time I don't recognize the vision of the person I see as anyone I know. Am I crazy?" Jada asked. "Am I really sending healing to others and helping them?"

Although Jada had several years of healing experience, distance healing can spontaneously occur for those who desire to help and heal others. Even though all types are able to send healing energy, spiritual intuitives may have the easiest time perceiving the energy field and tuning in to the presence of many varied vibrational levels of energy.

After learning more about the different medical intuitive types, you may discover that there is a bit of each one within you. You might instead feel comfortably familiar with one or two types. Either way, as you learn more about medical intuition, you will expand beyond your innate type and intuit through all four modalities. In the next chapter you will learn more about the natural psychic potential of each type.

8

THE FIVE BASIC MEDICAL INTUITIVE SKILLS

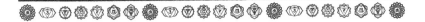

There are five basic psychic skills that form the foundation for medical intuitive ability. These five intuitive skills can be used to access energy information in many different areas of interest and concern. However, there are a few slightly different ways to develop and refine these abilities for use in medical intuition.

These five medical intuitive skills are clairvoyance, clairsentience, clairaudience, claircognizance, and vibrational sensitivity. Each of these skills corresponds with one or more of the intuitive types. Once you discover the way that you naturally intuit you will be able to develop and refine the natural strengths of your type and then build on this to develop the other psychic skills.

EXERCISE: CLAIRVOYANCE

Clairvoyance is the ability to visually see energy information. This may emerge in the form of literal and accurate three dimensional images. Clairvoyant images can also be more symbolic and figurative in nature. Although all of the intuitive types can develop clairvoyance, it often comes more naturally to spiritual intuitives.

At times clairvoyance may occur as spontaneous images that give information about your health or the health and well-being of another.

If you are naturally clairvoyant in this way, you can further refine this skill to view and gain understanding of the health of the physical body. However, this is a skill that can be learned with a little effort and practice. Either way, it is one of the most important psychic skills to develop, refine, and improve accuracy.

Because a significant aspect of medical intuition utilizes images to perceive and understand energy information, take the time needed to practice and build your confidence in this area. As you consistently use clairvoyance when scanning the physical and subtle energy body, perceiving energy information through images becomes more natural and instinctive.

Realistic Images

Through clairvoyant sight, images of the body organs and other systems often surface realistically and true to life. These images are often magnified and focused on an important and particular health issue or aspect. The colors in these images also tend to be true to life, the most predominant of which are usually red, blue, and whitish gray, and sometimes brown or black. It is common to see an image but not fully understand the significance of it, even when it is a realistic-looking image. When this happens you can tune in to it through the other intuitive skills and receive more energy information.

Figurative and Symbolic Images

Images that describe emotions, beliefs, and thought patterns will emerge more symbolically and figuratively. For instance, in a recent scan I became aware of a knot and pain in my client's right foot. I asked for an image of it and I saw raw, swollen tissue around a dry and chaffing bone. I described the image to my client and she confirmed that she had been experiencing a problem and pain in her foot. I then saw an image of my client with a man who I felt was her husband or partner. He was much taller and larger and loomed over her in a surreal cartoon-like way. As he did this she froze like a statue or a frozen block of ice. From this image I knew that she was emotionally frozen and intimidated. When I described the image to her, she told me that she wanted to move forward in her career but her husband was not supportive of her going back to work. Not knowing what to do, she told me that she felt unable to move forward. The pain in her foot was the physical manifestation of her feeling powerless to follow through with her desires.

FEELING AND THINKING CLAIRVOYANCE

Although this may seem hard to fully comprehend, sometimes clairvoyant perception occurs through more of an inner knowing, feeling, or sensation than a clear visual image. For instance, it is quite common for people to scan their energy field or body and have an intuitive sense of the color surrounding it without actually seeing it. Mental intuitives usually will know what the colors are. This is an instinctive sense of knowing, without full awareness of how they came to this conclusion. Emotional intuitives feel the colors. Each color has a particular feeling that can be difficult to put into words. Physical intuitives often have a sense of an image. This may be a gut sensation of sureness or a more visceral impression. However clairvoyant images emerge for you, trust what you experience and let it unfold.

At times throughout this book, you will be asked to use your imagination to perceive an image. Your imagination is a tool that your intuition uses to describe energy information to you in a way that you will understand and makes sense. Trust this process. As you become more comfortable with using clairvoyance, the difference between accessing energy information through imagination and images and purely making something up will become more apparent.

Do not block intuitive impressions because you expect them to appear to you in a certain way. Everyone intuits in a unique way. Discover yours and you will always be able to rely on it.

Try this: Close your eyes and take a deep, long, relaxing breath. Allow an image to emerge that represents your present state of health.

Use your imagination. You may see an image of yourself healthy and strong and engaged in a positive activity or an image that is cloudy and lacks energy. You might see a symbol, a cartoonlike figure, images of nature or uplifting scenes, or you may see colors and light. You may receive many different images or symbols and it is also possible that only one image slowly emerges.

Accept whatever you receive without trying to change or modify it.

EXERCISE: CLAIRSENTIENCE

Clairsentience provides both the ability to detect imbalances in the physical body and to uncover the underlying emotional causes of pain and illness. All of the intuitive types experience some form of clairsentience, but emotional and physical intuitives are the most likely to naturally use the psychic skill of clairsentience.

Physical intuitives experience clairsentience as visceral sensation in the body, usually in their solar plexus or in their hands, or they may feel the pain and illness of others in their physical body. Physical intuitives are the most likely to unknowingly absorb the physical aches and pains of others. The stomach or backache that abruptly emerges after sitting in a highly attended meeting all day and suddenly disappears when you are home may be energy that has been absorbed from another. The ability to sense the physical condition of another is a useful medical intuitive skill. Once you are aware that you are able to intuit energy information in this way, you can more quickly become conscious of what you are receiving and cease unknowingly absorbing others' energy into your body.

Emotional intuitives experience clairsentience more through emotion and feeling than physical sensation. Emotional intuitives are especially adept at uncovering the emotional triggers and the underlying emotional causes of pain and illness. They are often able to feel the traumatic and repressed feelings of others that may be at the root source of a physical health problem. This sometimes happens unexpectedly and it can cause confusion when you do not know what to do with this kind of sensitive intuitive information. An emotional intuitive might also intuitively feel the anger and resentment of a loved one and know that these feelings are creating the headaches and acid reflux that they are experiencing. If this has ever happened to you, you know the importance of understanding your innate intuitive nature and not taking on the emotions of others.

Many people receive personal health messages through clairsentience. I have had quite a few clients tell me that they have pursued getting a health checkup after experiencing strong feelings that something was not right with their health.

Clairsentience is a useful skill for the medical intuitive. It enables you to tune in to and feel emotional energy and the effect that it is having on the physical body. It also empowers you to sense and feel the health and condition of the body's organs and other physical systems.

Try this: Close your eyes and take a deep breath. Scan your body and notice any area that feels sore or tense or tight. Focus your awareness on one of these areas. Imagine that this area has an emotion connected to it. What is it? If this area had a texture, what would it feel like?

EXERCISE: CLAIRAUDIENCE

The ability to hear energy information is called clairaudience. Intuitive hearing may occur externally or internally. Have you ever heard your name being called? Yet, you looked all around and there was no one present. This is external clairaudient hearing. Internal hearing is similar but its source is clearly from within. Have you ever heard an inner phrase repeated over and over or heard an inner voice speaking to you? Clairaudience can be an inner still small voice, a voice that sounds like your own or in the case of medical intuition, the energy of the body speaking to you.

Clairaudience occurs most naturally in mental and physical intuitives. Most mental intuitives carry on internal conversations with an inner voice. Although they usually believe the source of this inner voice to be their own thinking mind, quite often they are conversing with someone in the spirit realm or with energy information. Physical intuitives experience clairaudience more as an outer voice. Many physical intuitives can communicate with crystals, animals, and plants. Although they do not necessarily hear these things speak to them through outer hearing, the quiet inner voice they perceive seems to emanate from an external source. Many physical intuitives are also able to communicate with the body itself. The organs and bodily systems seem to speak to them or they hear messages about their health or the health of others.

Quite often during a medical intuitive session you will be given information by your client's loved ones in spirit, an angel, or a spirit helper. It is not always necessary to know the source of the information. The information itself is what is most important. Sometimes you will hear a word repeated over and over. Other times you may hear a concise explanation of a medical problem.

You may also hear a word or phrase over and over that you do not understand during a medical intuition session. If this happens, write the word down and look it up after the session.

Try this: Close your eyes and take a deep, cleansing breath. Like the exercise for clairsentience, scan your body and notice any area that feels sore or tense or tight. Focus your awareness on one of these areas. Imagine that this area has a voice and can communicate to you. What is it saying?

Exercise: Claircognizance

Claircognizance is the ability to intuitively know energy information. You may not know how you know, but you know. This type of intuitive insight may be the most common psychic ability. When we spontaneously receive intuitive insights in this way, it may seem so easy that we often discount it. Most people intuitively know more about their physical health then they admit and acknowledge, even to themselves. Many people who get medical intuitive readings from me tell me that they have come in for a session because they have a nagging sense that something is not "right." They may even know exactly what organ or bodily system is in need of healing, but they do not totally trust their intuitive knowing. Quite often clients have been to a physician and everything has checked out fine. Still, they have an inner intuitive sense that pushes them to continue to investigate an undetected health problem. The body is wise and always communicating to you. Trust it. Those who do are usually grateful that they listened and acted on what they received.

In medical intuitive work, claircognizance plays an important role. It is often the glue that brings the images, colors in the energy field, and your intuited feelings and sensations into a comprehensive and full understanding. For instance, in intuitive body scans you may not always visualize an organ or other bodily system. Instead, you may have an intuitive sense of knowing what the organ looks like, along with other significant information. It can take a few trial and error attempts to become aware of when your intuitive knowing is correct and when it may not be connected to energy information. Clairsentience and claircognizance can work together quite well to help you to better know if what you are receiving is legitimate intuitive energy information. Through clairsentience many can feel the accuracy of energy information as an inner sensation and feeling of correctness and solid, calm certainty.

Claircognizance is primarily an intuitive talent of the mental intuitive. Yet, all of the types use the intuitive sense of knowing. Emotional intuitives often feel that they know the origins of emotional wounds and their effect on physical health. Many physical intuitives can place their hands on an individual or look at a photo and know where there is pain or problems. Spiritual intuitives experience claircognizance as the ability to know the meaning behind the clairvoyant images that easily come to them.

Try this: Close your eyes and breathe a deep, long, relaxing breath. Continue to breathe and relax.

Quiet your mind through gentle breaths. Ask yourself what you need to know about your health. Continue to breathe and receive whatever information comes to you.

Exercise: Vibrational Sensitivity

Although less known and practiced, the psychic skill of vibrational sensitivity is one that you will use quite a bit in medical intuitive sessions. The ability to sense energy flow and its density and rate of movement can reveal and uncover energy information that the other intuitive skills have a harder time accessing.

Although the physical body appears to be a solid mass, it is a dense form of energy. Medical intuitive readings are essentially the ability to tune in to energy flow, movement, and mass, and discern and interpret its energetic content. Vibrational sensitivity empowers you to tune in to the energy information contained in the body, chakras, meridians, and the aura. All of the four intuitive types use the psychic skill of vibrational sensitivity, although it comes most naturally to the physical intuitive.

Emotional intuitives tune in to the emotional energetic layer of the subtle energy body. In this layer of energy they are able to feel the lighter vibration energy currents of positive and love-infused energy. They are also able to feel the more dense and stifled flow of repressed and blocked emotional wounds and negative emotions.

Mental intuitives are attuned to the mental energetic layer in the subtle body. In this layer of energy they are able to feel the heightened flow of wisdom and positive thoughts from divine source energy and the lower vibration thoughts of negativity and judgment. Like the emotional intuitives, they are also able to detect the energetic blocks that develop when we constantly engage in negative and fear-based thoughts.

Spiritual intuitives are aligned with spiritual energy. They are able to vibrationally access higher and more complex levels of cosmic energy. As medical intuitives, they are able to intuit these cosmic vibrations as they move and flow through the physical body—nurturing, healing, and revitalizing it. They are also able to detect when the flow of source energy is being stifled, blocked, or cut off. Spiritual intuitives also utilize the skill of vibrational sensitivity to tune in to the energy field and the subtle body.

Physical intuitives are attuned to the denser vibrations of energy that soon manifest as physical matter. Unlike the spiritual intuitives, they tend to focus on the flow of energy through the physical body. Every organ and system of the body depends on energy movement for its health and well-being. The circulatory, nervous, endocrine, digestive, and all other systems maintain health in part by movement, interaction, and interconnectedness.

In perfect health we are a flowing high-vibration current of energy. When this flow of energy ceases, becomes blocked, or cut off from source energy or hindered in movement, we become imbalanced and eventually ill. For these reasons, the psychic skill of vibrational sensitivity is vital to intuiting health and well-being.

Try this: Sit next to a flowing river or stand outside on a windy day. Close your eyes and imagine that you can merge with the energy flow. Feel the vibration of the flow of the water in the river or the wind. Imagine that you can adjust your inner vibration to match that of the natural elements. Another way to tune in to vibrational sensitivity is to put both of your hands on the trunk of a large tree, a rock, or in the sunlight and sensitize yourself to the vibrational flow of these and other natural elements.

In the next section you will put the five basic medical intuitive skills to work, tuning in to your physical and subtle body. Remember the intuitive guidelines included in this chapter and refer back to them as often as necessary.

Section 3

RESIDENCY: DEVELOPING MEDICAL INTUITIVE SKILLS

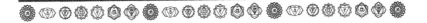

THE PHYSICAL BODY:
THE INTUITIVE VIEW

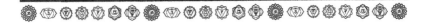

In this section you are invited to further explore the psychic skills, learn about the subtle body, the aura, the meridians, and the chakras.

This chapter provides you with the opportunity to develop and practice intuitively tuning in to your physical body. The following exercises better familiarize you with the psychic skills of clairvoyance, clairsentience, clairaudience, claircognizance, and vibrational sensitivity. These skills empower you to access and receive health and well-being energy information. Depending on your natural intuitive type, some of these exercises will come easier to you than others.

Begin by finding a quiet place where you will not be disturbed. Have a tape recorder or a journal close by to take notes. Do as much of this exercise as you can do until you begin to feel tired. You can continue where you left off in another practice session.

EXERCISE: CLAIRVOYANCE: CLEAR SEEING

Clairvoyance is the ability to see energy information, either figuratively or in a realistic and accurate three-dimensional form.

Take a deep breath; send the breath through the body. Relax and exhale any stress and tension though the outbreath. Continue this relaxing, cleansing breath.

Focus on your stomach and continue breathing. Fill your abdomen with breath; relax and exhale. Notice your abdomen fill as you breathe, then release as you exhale. Continue inhaling in this manner and exhaling, letting go of any tension and stress.

When you feel as if you are relaxed, make the intention to see within your abdomen. Intend to see your stomach. As you breathe, repeat this statement several times: "My intention is to see the energy of my stomach. I would like to see the energy of my stomach."

Continue to breathe and repeat this statement. You may want to close your eyes or keep them open. Try this both ways. Clairvoyance can manifest as outer sight or inner sight. With outer sight, you are able to visually see the energy of your stomach, almost as a superimposed image over or within the body. Inner sight is a bit different. With your eyes closed, imagine a blank screen. It may at first feel as if you are using your imagination to create an image. Go with this. Your imagination is a clairvoyant tool that empowers you to visually see. On this screen ask to see the energy of your stomach. You can again use your imagination. Notice the color or colors of this energy and any other detail that strikes you. Some people will see the stomach in a realistic form. Others will see the energy of the stomach as color and energy vibration. Either way is fine. Accept what surfaces and trust your intuitive style.

Keep in mind that each intuitive will experience clairvoyance differently. Emotional intuitives may feel a visual image of the stomach. A mental intuitive may know the visual image, physical intuitives may see a more realistic vision of the stomach organ, and spiritual intuitives may see a more abstract image.

As you repeat this exercise your clairvoyant ability will increase and strengthen.

EXERCISE: CLAIRSENTIENCE: INTUITIVE FEELING

Clairsentience is the psychic ability to intuit feeling and feeling sensation, either as an emotion or as a visceral and more physical feeling of mass, texture, and size.

Once you have clairvoyantly tuned in with your stomach:

Take a deep breath; send the breath through the body. Relax and exhale any stress and tension through the outbreath. Continue this relaxing, cleansing breath.

When you are relaxed make the intention to feel your stomach.

"My intention is to feel the energy of my stomach. I would like to now feel the energy of my stomach." Continue to breathe and repeat this statement.

You can now either tune in to the clairvoyant image of your stomach from the first part of this exercise or focus on the energy of the stomach. Ask to intuitively feel your stomach mass, and tune in to its depth, size, and texture.

Take your time. Write down or record whatever sensations and feelings you experience.

Take a deep breath—a long exhale—and relax. Focus your attention on your stomach and ask to clairvoyantly see an image of it.

Imagine that within and surrounding your stomach you can sense emotion. What is the predominant emotion or feeling connected to your stomach? Pay attention to any feelings that emerge.

Emotional intuitives may readily feel an emotion connected to the stomach and have a more difficult time feeling it as texture, mass, and size. Mental intuitives may intuit both the emotion connected to the stomach and its mass and size through a sense of knowing. A physical intuitive may tune in to the emotion as a gut feeling or sense of knowing while having an easier time intuiting the stomach's size, texture, and mass. A spiritual intuitive may see or sense emotion as color and might also intuit the texture and size of the stomach through a more figurative image.

Take your time and write down whatever feelings emerge.

As you repeat this exercise your clairsentient ability will increase.

Exercise: Clairaudience: Sixth Sense Hearing

Clairaudience is the ability to hear energy information either through inner or outer hearing. This exercise gives you the opportunity to begin to communicate and dialogue with energy. This is an important skill that you will use in the medical intuitive body scans.

Take a deep breath and send the energy of the breath through the body. Relax and exhale any stress and tension through the outbreath. Continue this relaxing, cleansing breath.

When you are relaxed make the intention to listen to and hear the energy of your stomach.

"My intention is to hear the energy of my stomach. I would like to now listen to the energy of my stomach." Continue to breathe and repeat this statement.

Intuitively tune in to a clairvoyant image of the energy of your stomach. Remember this can be a visual image that you perceive through outer or inner sight. You may perceive the energy superimposed over the body or on a blank screen image. Feel the texture and tune in to the color of the energy.

Imagine that your stomach has a voice and can speak to you. What is it saying? Quietly listen. You may hear requests to eat certain foods and avoid others. Your stomach may also communicate that all is well or it may inform you of a need to breathe, relax, and release stress. Let go of any expectation of what your stomach may or may not communicate to you. Just listen. Remember you may not hear your stomach as an audible voice. It may instead feel as if you are hearing this in your head as your thoughts, or in your own voice.

Emotional intuitives may intuitively hear the emotional energy of the stomach. Mental intuitives may hear the energy information more through inner hearing, almost as if they are simply talking to themselves. A physical intuitive may easily tune in to the physical stomach but not be able to hear it speak. If this is the case, imagine that the stomach has a voice and can speak to you. Then listen to what it is saying. A spiritual intuitive may see a more clairvoyant colorful image. If this is the case, ask the color to communicate to you.

As you repeat this exercise your clairaudience ability will increase.

EXERCISE: VIBRATIONAL SENSITIVITY: SENSING THE FLOW

Vibrational sensitivity is the ability to intuit energy flow, movement, and vibration. This is an important medical intuitive skill.

Take a deep breath; send the breath through the body. Relax and exhale any stress and tension though the outbreath. Continue this relaxing, cleansing breath.

When you are relaxed make the intention to tune in to the energy flow of the stomach.

Repeat the statement. "My intention is to tune in to the energy flow of my stomach. I would like to now intuit the vibrational energy flow of my stomach." Continue to breathe and repeat this statement.

Intuitively tune in to a clairvoyant image of the energy of your stomach. This can be a visual image that you perceive through outer or inner sight. You may perceive the energy superimposed over the body or as an inner screen image. Tune in to the color of energy and feel its flow.

Emotional intuitives may intuit flow as feeling and emotion moving through the body. A mental intuitive is likely to know the flow. Physical and spiritual intuitives may have the easiest time feeling vibrational movement. However you initially experience this, keep stating your intent to feel the vibration of energy. Pause and receive.

When there is a dysfunction, imbalance, illness, or any concern about an organ or bodily system you will be alerted by the sensation of a tingle, the lighting up of an image, or the feeling of a hard knot, an inert stagnant area, or an erratic uneven flow of energy. Pay attention to these kinds of vibrational occurrences. They signal a problem. If the energy is flowing smoothly without interruption and feels somewhat flat, this is a positive sign. If your intent is to intuit problem areas and illness, energy will get your attention through noticeable energy flow interruptions.

Once you tune in to the energy flow of your stomach, imagine the energy as color. Notice if it is luminous and radiant or if it is shaded and dull. Healthy energy will be light and flow evenly.

Write down or record your experiences.

EXERCISE: CLAIRCOGNIZANCE: PSYCHIC KNOWING

Claircognizance is the ability to intuitively know. You may not know how you know, but you know. Our organs and bodily systems contain an energy layer of mental energy. Within this energy are our beliefs, thoughts, and attitudes. These thoughts and beliefs affect our health and well-being. Claircogniznce is the ability to tune in to this mental layer of energy. This is often experienced as a full and complete awareness that is not linear, but complex energy information that suddenly emerges.

Take a deep breath; send the breath through the body. Relax and exhale any stress and tension through the outbreath. Continue this relaxing, cleansing breath.

Intuitively tune in to a clairvoyant image of the energy of your stomach. This can be a visual image that you perceive through outer or inner sight. You may perceive the energy superimposed over the body or you may see an image of the energy of the stomach on an inner blank screen. Feel the texture and tune in to the color of the energy.

When you are relaxed make the intention to tune in to the thought energy of your stomach.

Make the statement. "My intention is to tune in to the mental energy layer of my stomach. I would like to now know more about the thought energy stored in my stomach." Continue to breathe and repeat this statement.

Continue to breathe and become aware of your thoughts without becoming overly attached to any one thought. Intuitive thoughts have a consistent and calm quality. They return over and over in the same detached yet steady manner. Mind chatter incites emotion and can make you feel unsettled or excited. Intuitive thoughts are more matter-of-fact. You will also have an intuitive sense of their truth. Be aware that the ego mind may try to diagnose an illness or disease and likely give you names like cancer, diabetes, etc. Be cautious of this kind of information that is not backed up by energy, color, and vibration.

In addition, pay attention to the awareness of any beliefs, thoughts, and attitudes that may be negatively impacting your stomach or your digestive process.

Emotional intuitives may feel simultaneous intuitive insight into both mental and emotional energy. Mental intuitives may intuit more clear energy information. A physical intuitive may receive mental energy as a gut knowing, and spiritual intuitives may spontaneously receive information as to life purpose and past life influences.

Claircognizance can also be useful at the end of a body scan or as you move from one area of the body to another.

Take a deep breath; send the breath through the body. Relax and exhale any stress and tension though the outbreath. Continue this relaxing, cleansing breath.

When you are relaxed make the intention to receive intuitive information about your stomach.

Say within: "My intention is to receive energy information about my stomach. I would like to now receive energy information about my stomach." Continue to breathe and repeat this statement.

While doing this exercise you may receive visual, auditory, kinesthetic, and emotional energy information. You may receive many or just a few images, feelings, visual colors, and auditory information. Accept everything that you intuitively receive.

Claircognizance is the intuitive skill that empowers you to inuit what energy information is valid and usable and what information to disregard.

Make the intention to correctly discern the intuitive information that you have just received. "My intention is to know and correctly interpret what I have intuitively received. I would now like to know what is important and if my interpretation is correct." Repeat this statement.

Ask to review one piece of energy information at a time. Imagine a blank screen. Ask to see the first information that you received. As this image emerges, trust your inner knowing as to its accuracy. If the image is important it will not fade until you fully understand it. Once it fades you have made the correct determination. Then move on to the next information that you received. Repeat until you have gone through all that you have previously intuited. Now ask if there is anything else that you need to know. You can use your clairvoyant, clairsentience, clairaudience, claircognizance, and vibrational sensitivity skills to intuit any additional energy information.

Write down or record all that you experience.

X-Ray Intuitive Vision

Medical intuitive readings differ from other types of intuitive work in that the physical body is the defined focus of the session. However, it is important to remember that even though the physical body appears to be solid and finite, it is not. The body is the doorway to multidimensional and infinite energy. It is a complex and intelligent expression of cosmic and earthly energy. Expect the unexpected. Broaden your view of the kind of information that you receive. Don't go into a medical intuitive reading only focusing on the physical problems. To heal and help others to heal at the core level where illness and pain begin, be aware of any and all influences that surface. Do not ignore or discount the importance of any emotions, thoughts, past experiences, memories, and spiritual information that you intuit.

X-Ray intuitive vision is the ability to "see" within the physical body. However, intuition allows us to "see" in several different ways. Intuitive sight encompasses clairvoyance, clairsentience, claircognizance, vibrational sensitivity, and even clairaudience. From a three-dimensional perspective it is only possible to visually see with the eyes. However, intuitive seeing is an inner seeing that focuses on receiving and interpreting energy in whatever form it emerges. In medical intuitive body scans you will use the combination of all types of intuitive skills to perceive, receive, and understand energy information.

Congratulations! After having completed these exercises you are well on your way to using your intuition to tune in to the physical body. You may not feel especially intuitively adept yet. But you are further along than you might think. Be patient with yourself and the process. When you least expect it, it will all come together for you.

The following chapter will introduce you to the finer energy vibrations of the energy body and help you to use the psychic skills to tune in to this important aspect of your health and wellness.

10

THE AURA AND THE MERIDIANS: RAINBOWS OF ENERGY INFORMATION

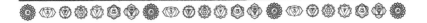

To develop medical intuition it is important to understand and form a relationship with energy. Every day in innumerable ways you consciously and unconsciously communicate with energy. As you become more aware of the dynamics of energy you will learn how to better intuitively communicate with it and receive valuable and important information.

Energy is the pure, pulsating, indestructible, creative essence that permeates all of life. It is everywhere and is within all things. It is the energy within the planets and the space surrounding them that keeps our physical existence balanced in perfect harmony. It is the energy within the silent seed that pushes it up from the dark ground and it is energy that pushes air into our lungs and keeps our heart beating. At our core, we, along with all living beings, are comprised of energy.

Given the solid appearance of our physical body it may not always be readily apparent, but you are a vibrating network of magnificent dancing energy. Like a swarm of birds sailing through the skies in perfect unison, or a school of tropical fish moving as one mind and one soul colorfully through the seas, our body, mind, and spirit interrelate and interact and move as one energetic force of being. When I tune in to the physical body of another I see this beauty. While looking in the mirror in the morning my client may have noticed a new wrinkle or stepped on the scale only to be dismayed that they have gained a pound. When I look at my clients, I instead see a maze of colorful energy.

My ability to perceive others as a colorful energy light show spontaneously occurred when I was about seventeen years old. I was playing volleyball with a group of friends. It was a gorgeous summer day. The green grass seemed more vibrant than usual and a nearby river sparkled in the sunlight. Suddenly, I saw bursts of color swirling and surrounding my friends. Awestruck by this unexpected display of energy and color, I stood staring at the incredible beauty in what felt like a moment stuck in time. As the colors eventually began to fade, I was hopeful that I would always be able to see others in this way. From a young age I have been able to see the colorful aura that surrounds plants and trees, but the energy that I was now seeing was unlike anything that I had previously experienced.

I am fortunately still able to see the wondrous orchestra of color, movement, and organized energy around others. For a time the ability to perceive energy around others came and went without my being able to control it. I am now able to activate my ability to see energy when I wish to and to tune in to the important energy information that it contains.

As attractive as the physical body may be, at our core we are a Technicolor, vibrant light show. Your physical body is a dense form of colorful energy vibration. Your mind and emotions are a less dense form of energy vibration, while your spirit vibrates to a much higher frequency. We are blood, bones, muscle, and tissue governed by a vast web of intelligence, love, and cosmic vibration that extends from the higher realms of light energy to the dense manifestations of matter.

The pulsating and colorful network of energy that surrounds our physical body is referred to as our subtle energy body. Many different spiritual traditions throughout time have identified it and understood it to be the gateway through which the soul interacts with the higher spiritual planes and the physical body. It has been referred to as the "most sacred body" in Sufism, the "body of bliss" in Kriya Yoga, "the light body" or "rainbow body" in Tibetan Buddhism, the "diamond body" in Taoism, and "the immortal body" in Hermeticism.

For the medical intuitive the subtle energy body cannot be separated from the physical body. They are one and the same. Together they contain vital and important energy information through which you can gain valuable insight into the mental, emotional, spiritual, and physical health and well-being of an individual. Within the subtle energy body are points of power and wisdom that you can tune in to. These power points are the aura, the meridians, and the chakras. They are the spiritual and physical entry points through which vital life force source energy is transmitted to the physical, emotional, and mental levels of being. For a medical intuitive the subtle body reveals all truths.

The Aura

The aura is the outermost egg-shaped web of energy surrounding the physical body. It is comprised of pulsating energy vibration and color that expands and contracts with graceful fluidity. The aura is made up of seven inner layers of energy, each serving a specific function. These energy layers are the interface between the physical body and cosmic life force source energy. Each layer of the aura serves an important evolutionary spiritual and physical function.

The first layer is called the etheric level or etheric body. It is shaped like your physical body and located about two inches from it. This is the easiest layer of the aura to intuitively perceive. The etheric body holds physical health energy information. When you intuitively tune in to this layer of energy you can become aware of current physical health issues and soon-to-manifest health issues.

The emotional, creative layer of the aura surrounds the etheric layer. It is about three inches from the body. In this layer of energy it is possible to intuitively tune in to an individual's ability to harness the power of their emotional and creative energy to materially manifest. The colors of this layer give insight into an individual's range of emotions and manifestation energy.

The third layer of the aura is the mental layer. It is about three to eight inches from the body. This layer is infused with the ever-evolving balance between the higher soul self and the personality self, one's thoughts, and personal power.

The astral layer extends about a foot from the physical body. It is the doorway through which you can access spiritual energy and the astral plane. It draws in energy from the spirit realm and infuses the mental, emotional, and physical layers with vital life force energy fuel.

The etheric template is the next layer. It extends up to two feet from the body. This template holds all the possibilities that you can draw from over the course of your life. This layer does not usually change during a lifetime but it can evolve. The manifestation possibilities inherent in the etheric template are dependent on the overall health of the previous layers. Negative emotions, critical limited thoughts and judgments, and emotional wounds limit the potential absorption of this layer into the physical experience.

The celestial aura or sixth layer extends about two and a half feet from the physical body. It is through this layer that we connect with the angelic realm, spirit helpers, and divine beings. The celestial aura is also connected to the higher vibrations of love, bliss, inspiration, and joy. When you are in alignment with this field you feel a cosmic oneness with all of life. There is nothing that you can do that will alter or change the celestial layer. At any time you can draw from it for wisdom, guidance, and cosmic love.

The seventh layer of the aura is the ketheric template or life force layer. It can extend to over three feet from the body. It surrounds all of the other layers and holds them together. It vibrates to the highest frequency and contains all of your soul experiences throughout many lives, your present life plan, and the ultimate destiny and individuality of your spirit. This is your connection to the divine.

Each of the seven layers filters and regulates the interaction and interconnectedness between an individual's spiritual, mental, emotional, and physical energy. The aura also protects the body from toxins and unbeneficial energies and acts as an antenna to attract positive and life-giving pure energy.

Detecting the Condition of the Aura

The aura communicates intuitive energy information primarily through color and vibration. When intuitively tuning in to the aura begin by feeling its size, strength, general form, and condition. A healthy aura is luminous and flowing. You can feel and sometimes hear its vibration like a gentle humming. Pay attention to the range of colors, their quality and shade, and more importantly, where in the aura these colors emanate from.

A damaged aura is dull, too small or too large, and has holes and/or tears. These conditions indicate an existing or soon-to-manifest dysfunction or illness in the physical body. People who have endured long-term drug or alcohol addiction, childhood abuse, or emotional, mental, physical, or spiritual trauma are most at risk of having a damaged aura. In addition, some children have oversized or unformed auras. This almost always is caused by conflict between the soul and the present physical incarnation. A soul may be resisting the life script that it has been born into or it may miss the freedom and expansiveness of living in the spirit realm. A misshaped aura in children usually manifests as food and environmental allergies, hyperactivity, problems with sleep, learning disabilities, and oversensitivity to noise and physical stimulation and similar issues that can be difficult to diagnose and heal.

For instance, during the course of a session that I had with Rebecca, a mother of three young children, she asked me about her son David's health.

I said to her, "I am feeling a lot of congestion in his sinuses and lungs. It feels as if he has allergies. He is very sensitive; noise and light can bother him."

"He has chronic allergies and yes, he is very sensitive. Everything seems to bother him—noise, smells, and food. I don't know what to do. I have taken him to several specialists, but the medication they prescribe seems to cause more problems," she said. "I have tried everything and I don't know where to go from here."

As I continued to intuitively tune in to David's energy to better understand the root of his problem, I was drawn to his aura. It was dull and shapeless. Above his head there was an opening and it looked as if his aura had not fully formed. He had no energetic protection; toxins and disruptive energy were pouring into his overwhelmed system.

"Your son was reluctant to be born into this present life. His soul wanted to maintain a connection with the divine realms and it is using the opening in his aura as a misguided escape hatch. It is important to talk to your son and reinforce the idea that he came into this life to experience joy and happiness. I know it might seem that he is too young to fully understand this, but there is a part of him that needs to hear this over and over. A spiritual connection of some kind is also very important. It does not have to be a church or organized group. Being in nature, reading books for children about angels and spirituality and making sure he gets fresh air and sunshine will help," I shared with her.

"David is a very spiritually attuned child. He tells me about his dreams and the spirit people that talk to him. He once told me it was a mistake that he was here. He said he wanted to go back to the angels. I told him that I loved him and he was meant to be my son," Rebecca explained.

"David is in a little boy body, but he is an old soul. He has a purpose and mission for being here at this time. He wanted to be done with his earth lives, but he came back to help others. You might want to help him remember this. Your son's aura needs a little encouragement to come into full vitality. Every day you can visualize in your mind's eye a strong and resilient orb of protective light completely surrounding him. Ask his angels to cover him in light and shield him."

I saw Rebecca several months later. She told me that after our session, David seemed to have good days and bad days. Although he seemed more present in his body, and his allergies were improving, he seemed to be unsettled. She eventually sat him down and told him that there was an important reason he was here in the physical world.

"What is it?" he asked her.

"I'm not sure, but I know you came to help others in some way. I also know that you are a special boy and your angels are watching over you," she told him.

"I know I can feel them close. I didn't know that you could see them too," he excitedly said.

Rebecca continued to talk to him about his angels and his purpose. She told me that a calm feeling of peace seemed to come over him. Since then they have talked about angels several times.

"He is doing so much better now," she told me. "He is playing with his brother and sister more, enjoying running around outdoors, and seems genuinely much happier. His allergies and other sensitivities are becoming less and less of a problem."

EXERCISE: DETECT THE AURA

The following exercise will empower you to better perceive the energy field or aura. Keep in mind that intuitively perceiving energy involves more than the physical eyes. Use your intuitive clairvoyant sight. It may feel like you are using your imagination and making up colors if you do not readily see them through physical sight. However, remember that your imagination is a tool that your intuition uses to interpret energy information.

Go to a dimly lit room and light a candle or go outside in the sunlight. Sit or lie down. Relax and inhale a long deep breath and exhale, releasing any stress and tension. Stretch your arms out and open your hands so that your palms are facing upright.

Breathe and tune in to energy vibration through your palms using the psychic skill of vibrational sensitivity. It may feel slightly tingly, warm, pulsating, or dense. You may detect a flow or current of energy moving through your palms. Take a few moments to tune in to any sensations.

Using the psychic skills of clairvoyance, tune in to the energy color emanating from your palms. Remember to tap into your intuition to "see" the energy. It is not only with the human eye but with inner sight, knowing, and feeling that we "see" energy. You may see one primary color that vanishes when you blink. You may also see a translucent colorless ring of energy or a shimmering glow. Be patient with this process. It may take practice to clearly feel and see the aura.

Continue to breathe and relax. Move your hands slowly toward you, pausing every inch or so or until you feel a shift in vibration and mass. Remember to use the psychic skill of vibrational sensitivity. When you pause, take a moment to feel the energy vibration. At some point as you move your hands toward your body you will feel a density or more rapid, increased flow of energy. These shifts in vibration are the different layers of your energy field. Using the psychic skills, tune in to the colors of your energy field.

Move your hands up and then down your body, staying in contact with the most tangible dense layer of energy that you encounter. Move your hands closer to the body, pausing every inch or so. Tune in to the range of colors and feel the varying vibrations of energy layers. Become aware of any places in the energy field where you feel abrupt changes or where the energy field may feel tight, misshapen, or irregular. If you come across these kinds of vibrational changes, pause, open both palms toward the area, and imagine sending love and healing energy to any place in your energy field that may need balancing and alignment.

When you have finished, draw the outline of a person on a white sheet of paper. With colored pencils or crayons draw the shape and colors of the aura that you just intuited.

You can also practice this exercise with another. Have a friend sit or lie down in a dimly lit room or outside. Begin by standing several feet away from him or her. Open your hands and have your palms face the person you are scanning. Walk slowly toward him or her until you feel a shift in the energy vibration. Most likely it will feel dense or tingly when you are in contact with their aura. Slowly move forward, inch by inch. Tune in to the energy vibration and color and shape of their aura. Record what you receive.

Meridians

Within the aura is a vast network of energy pathways called the meridians. They act as the body's energy "bloodstream," carrying energy to every organ and physiological system. The meridians move life force energy throughout the body, bring balance, and remove energy blockages. Acting as a uniting force of energy, meridians integrate the mind, body, and spirit into one being. There are fourteen meridians with twelve connecting segments. Each meridian corresponds with the organ they direct energy through, yet they act in unison as one flow of energy.

The fourteen major meridians are the central meridian, the governing meridian, the spleen meridian, the heart meridian, the small intestine meridian, the bladder meridian, the kidney meridian, the circulation-sex meridian, the triple warmer meridian, the gall bladder meridian, the liver meridian, the lung meridian, the large intestine meridian, and the stomach meridian. Meridians are essential to the health of the body. If blocked or unregulated, the body becomes sluggish and disease results.

Through X-Ray intuitive vision, which is using the five psychic skills in unison, meridians can be intuitively detected as colorful undulating streams of energy flowing up and down and through the many and varied systems of the body. They provide information about an individual's psychological and emotional energy, as well as insight into the condition and health of the organs and other bodily systems.

Ted came in for a session with me on the advice of his wife. Newly married, he lovingly agreed. I don't think that he so much wanted to have a reading as he wanted to be a good husband. In his late thirties, he was a handsome man who was well built and athletic. Ted was not sure what a session entailed. He told me that he had no particular questions or areas to explore.

"Just tell me what you get," he said.

I began the reading and shared the information that I received about his work and family, and I communicated with a few of his loved ones on the other side. Although he looked healthy and fit, I decided to scan his body. When I did this the meridian that ran through his heart caught my attention. I could feel its vibrant energy flow—until I came to his heart. As the meridian flowed over his heart I felt it speed up and jump. I scanned it a few times and every time I did the energy flow was interrupted in the same way.

"Your heart seems to be at risk of rapid and irregular beating," I told him.

"I have had a heart arrhythmia for several years," Ted shared with me. "The doctor thinks that it's congenital. I'm on medication for it."

Although the medication was keeping Ted's heartbeat regular, it was not altering the flow of energy through the heart meridian. Intuitively tuning in to the energy of the meridians can give an indication of what may manifest in a person's health. It also shows the importance of healing the emotional, mental, and spiritual issues underlying physical problems.

Ted's father was a successful attorney who had high expectations for his son. Ted was expected to excel in sports, academics, and later, in his career. As I tuned in to Ted's meridian and heart chakra I saw images of him when he was younger, stressed and anxious over his ability to make his father happy. I could feel a tight band of energy around his chest. The meridian that ran through his heart was constricted.

I shared what I received with Ted and he seemed surprised that I was able to know about both his heart condition and his young anxiety-ridden relationship with his father. As we talked I could feel him begin to relax and let go of this long-term unconscious stress. Before he left he assured me that he would continue to be mindful of his inner stress and even try practicing meditation.

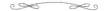

The aura and the meridians are more elusive to intuitively detect than the organs and many of the systems of the physical body. For most people it is best to initially focus on the psychic skills of vibrational sensitivity and clairvoyance to better tune in to them. The other psychic skills will naturally follow suit and provide you with more energy information.

The next chapter will introduce you to chakras—rich storehouses of energy information.

11

THE CHAKRAS:
SPIRALS OF LIFE

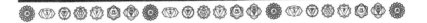

Chakras are spiral discs of energy that act as receivers and distributors of pure life force energy throughout the body. There are seven major chakras located from above the head to the base of the spine. These seven chakras are each encoded with seven varying levels of vibration that absorb and process our emotional, mental, spiritual, and physical experiences and life lessons. Each chakra contains a diary of information about our present and past life challenges, karma, and soul purpose and potential.

The health and vitality of the physical body directly correlates to the health of the chakras. Highly sensitive to our thoughts, actions, feelings, experiences, and spiritual purpose, the chakras are influenced and affected by all that we experience. While we can consciously deny our feelings, harbor negativity and critical judgments, stuff our pain away, and detach from our personal power, our chakras absorb all of this material. The chakras are never in denial. The heavier energy vibrations of negativity, pain, and powerlessness block and restrict the chakras from distributing the necessary flow of vital life force source energy to our organs and physiological systems. When vibrant source energy does not flow freely through the chakras, the physical body, tires, withers, and eventually becomes imbalanced and ill.

The chakras are a gold mine of intuitive information. Each of the seven chakras corresponds to specific organs and bodily functions. They contain intuitive information about the emotional, mental, and spiritual issues that contribute to disease, illness, pain, and dysfunction.

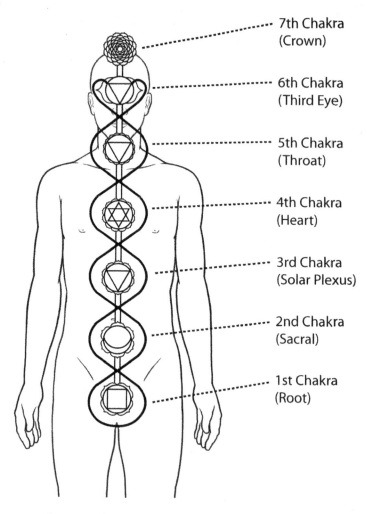

7th Chakra
(Crown)

6th Chakra
(Third Eye)

5th Chakra
(Throat)

4th Chakra
(Heart)

3rd Chakra
(Solar Plexus)

2nd Chakra
(Sacral)

1st Chakra
(Root)

Figure 1: The Seven Chakras

The Root Chakra

The first chakra is the root or base chakra. It is located at the base of the spine and its vibrational color is red. This power center is energetically coded with issues of survival, our sense of belonging, our instincts, and our ability to live our purpose. The function of this chakra is to empower us to fully live our divine purpose in the physical material world. When we are unable to identify and make choices that demonstrate our highest good in a concrete way this chakra loses its necessary energy fuel. We experience fear, insecurity, and lack the ability to take care of ourselves. The root chakra also connects us to the earth and to the people, animals, and living beings with whom we can enjoy a compatible relationship. Without a sense of authentic connection to others in the physical world, our soul becomes adrift with no anchor. The body loses energy as if it is a limb cut off from a tree.

The intuitive information contained in this chakra has to do with our early family issues and experiences, our ability to connect with others and the environment, and our capacity to move forward and make concrete changes in our everyday life. The organs and body systems related to the first chakra are the immune system, the blood, skeletal structure and bones, coccygeal nerve plexus, and the legs, feet, and rectum. The dysfunctions associated with this chakra are varicose veins, prostate problems, rectal and large intestine problems and tumors, depression, sciatica, hip, leg, and feet issues, frequent illness and immune-related disorders, anorexia, and obesity.

Food as Family

I gave a medical intuitive reading to Carol by phone. When I initially scanned her, I was drawn to her lower body. Even though I start a scan at the top of the head, my intuitive attention kept leading me to her left knee. When I asked for more information and images of the physical problem, I saw inflammation and deterioration around her kneecap.

"Your knee feels weak and swollen," I told Carol. "I feel a lot of inflammation and water retention in your calves and ankles."

"It's been like this off and on for a while," Carol confirmed. "It is getting harder and harder to get around."

As I continued to scan and ask questions of the energy I became aware of her weight. She was a large woman. Even though she was miles away I could see the extra weight she carried and could feel her embarrassment at being obese.

"It feels to me that you have some extra weight that is contributing to the weakness in your knees and water retention," I said.

Before I could finish Carol interrupted me.

"I know I am a big woman; been big all of my life. Doesn't help to diet, I have tried every one. I have about given up. So please don't lecture me about my weight. I have heard it all," she told me defensively.

I knew from her strong reaction that to help her I would have to approach her with compassion and understanding.

"Would it help if I looked at the root issue behind your struggles with weight?" I asked her.

"Yes, I would like to know this. Why can't I lose weight?" Carol responded.

With her request, I immediately saw an image of a little girl about seven years old. "I see a young girl with pretty curly blond hair sitting alone outside. I believe this is you. You are singing a song almost under your breath. I get the feeling of grief and a lot of deep sadness. It feels as if there has been a loss." As I shared this with Carol, I heard a faint cry come over the phone receiver. I stopped for a moment and Carol asked me to continue.

"Please go on," she said. "I haven't thought of this for a long time."

"There has been a passing. Did you have a younger sibling, a brother, who died as a baby?" I asked her.

"Yes, he died when he was just a few months old of a congenital heart problem. But I never really knew him. Could this be at the root of my problems with weight?"

"I feel that when you lost your brother, your only sibling, there was a tremendous amount of grief and loss in the environment," I shared with Carol. "You soaked this in. You felt your family fall apart and became confused and lost. You blamed yourself. It feels to me that your mother became depressed and despondent. Your father focused on work and became silent. You were alone."

"I was alone from then on," Carol shared with me. "Both of my parents drifted away. My father spent most of his time at work and one day he simply did not come home. My parents divorced and my mother started to drink during the day. I feel that I have been alone since that time. I have never been married and my only close friend died several years ago. I guess food has been my only comfort."

I continued the reading with Carol. She was much more receptive and willing to try to make some changes in her diet, and even seemed enthused with starting to exercise.

When we feel known and understood we feel connected. When I was able to intuit the core issue behind her weight problems, Carol no longer felt as if she was suffering in silence.

Exercise: Vibrational Sensitivity
and the First Chakra: Connect to Good Health

The following exercise will help you to tune in to the energy of your first chakra by tuning in to energy flow and vibration through the psychic skill of vibrational sensitivity.

Sit or lie down and breathe relaxing breaths. Focus your intuitive awareness at the base of your spine and tune in to the first chakra's circular flow of energy. You may want to place the palm of your hand a few inches from either the front or back of the lowest part of your torso.

Tune in to the energy vibration and flow of the first chakra.

Through the psychic skill of vibrational sensitivity get a sense of the health of this chakra. Does is it feel imbalanced, tight or loose, expanded or contracted?

Breathe energy into the first chakra and intend for this chakra to expand and come into balance. Take a few moments to feel the increase of energy moving through the chakra. With your hand a few inches from the lowest part of your torso feel the energy expand and contract through your palms.

With your eyes closed tune in to this chakra's vibration and flow and visualize a red spiral of energy. Imagine this chakra rooted in the earth. Like the roots of a tall tree, feel yourself anchored, grounded, and connected to the here and now. Breathe into the root chakra and feel the flow of vital life force energy of the earth move up through the body. Breathe down through the top of the head and feel the higher vibrations of cosmic life force energy move down through the body. Continue to breathe vital life force energy up through the root chakra and cosmic life force energy down from the top of the head. Feel your body flow with the energy of good health. Imagine every organ, bodily system, muscle, cell, and tissue absorbing healing life force energy.

Write down or draw anything that you feel, see, hear, know, and sense from this chakra.

The Sacral Chakra

The second chakra is the sacral chakra. It is located below the abdomen and vibrates to the color orange. This power center is concerned with our creativity, sexuality, our issues of control, and our learning how to harness our emotional and creative energy into material manifestation. This is the Johnny Appleseed of chakras as it empowers us to receive and spread the seeds of life force energy out into the material world. Give and take, sharing and receiving, producing and experiencing— this chakra teaches us balance.

Empowering us to draw from the well of cosmic energy within, the sacral chakra motivates us to make our way in the world. When we expect to be taken care of by others and do not draw from our inner authentic source energy, we negate the power of this chakra.

Compromising our authentic power in favor of unfulfilling relationships, unsatisfying work or career choices, and empty physical distractions and pleasure weakens the health of this chakra.

The intuitive information contained within this chakra includes issues of material success, finances, relationships, our ability to express and share our creativity and passions, and our ability to manifest our dreams. Issues with sexuality, reproduction, childbirth, and the ability to express physical and sexual intimacy can also be found in this chakra. Feelings of guilt, shame, and blame, the need to control others or allowing ourself to be controlled, and addictions are located in the second chakra.

The sacral chakra governs our spleen, sexual organs, liver, upper intestines, kidneys, gallbladder, adrenal glands, pancreas, and middle spine. Physical dysfunctions associated with this chakra are low back pain, fertility issues, ob/gyn problems, fibroids, uterine cysts, impotence, pelvic pain, libido, and urinary problems.

I Want to Have a Baby

One of the most common reasons that women seek medical intuitive readings is for issues with fertility, perimenopause, menopause, and difficulties with hormonal changes. When Claire came in for her session, she appeared to be full of energy and upbeat. Yet, despite her appearance I immediately felt an underlying feeling of stress and exhaustion. As I began the session I felt her mind running in circles. I knew that she did not sleep well and had not gotten a good night's sleep in quite a while.

"You have an active mind. It feels like you are not going into the deeper sleep cycles," I began.

"This is one of the reasons I'm here," Claire confirmed.

I attempted to continue to intuitively tune in to her issues with sleep, but kept feeling guided to her second chakra. I have learned over time not to try to override my natural intuitive impulses. I go where I am directed. As soon as I focused on the second chakra, I knew the primary reason for her visit with me.

"Claire, do you want to become pregnant?" I asked. "I am being drawn to your reproductive energy, and I feel a sadness and stress here."

"Yes, that's the other reason I'm here. My husband and I have been trying to get pregnant for months. But it's not happening."

"As I tune in to your ovulation and fallopian tubes I feel that there isn't enough energy juice for the spark of conception. I see them as dry and lifeless," I explained to Claire. "When I ask what you can do to create more of the necessary spark, I see an image of you in an office."

"I work in an office downtown," Claire responded.

"I am getting the impression that you do not feel connected to your job. You seem empty; like you're watching the clock and can't wait for the end of the day. It may not seem connected to you, but your dissatisfaction with work has, over time, created a very sterile and lifeless inner climate. To conceive you need to conjure up some authentic positive energy. Did you go to school for a different occupation; one that you felt passionate about?" I asked.

"I have a degree in fine arts, in photography. But, I can't make a living taking pictures. I work in accounts receivable. Not a job that I would have ever thought I would do. I always envisioned that I would be involved in more creative pursuits. My job is a dead end and I know it, but what am I supposed to do about it? I need the money," Claire told me.

"Your angels seem to have a message for you," I told her. "They say that it is important for you to incorporate your creative vision in some way in your day-to-day life. You cannot just wait for the perfect job to come your way. You have an amazing talent and life force energy. But you are squashing it. You must find an avenue for your creativity. It does not have to be a job right now. It can be a hobby or pastime and maybe this will develop into something else down the line. Right now, to conceive a baby, you must put more energy into you."

"You're kind of telling me what I've known for a while. I guess I just needed to have someone else confirm what I already know. I so much want to be more creative. I just thought that I was being selfish and that to be a good wife, and one day a mother, I had to put aside these crazy, creative ideas."

Claire seemed more alive just telling me this.

"It's not crazy. It's you. You cannot cut off a part of yourself and expect to thrive and conceive," I told her.

EXERCISE: CLAIRSENTIENCE AND THE
SECOND CHAKRA: YOUR EMOTIONS AND MANIFESTATION

This exercise will empower you to tune in to the emotional energy of your second chakra and further develop your ability to sense and feel emotional energy within the body. You will use the psychic skill of clairsentience.

Sit or lie down and breathe relaxing breaths. Focus your intuitive awareness about an inch below your abdomen. With the psychic skill of vibrational sensitivity feel the circular flow of energy of the second chakra. Imagine that this chakra pulls energy up from the first chakra and down from the higher chakras. This energy flows out into the world, manifesting in such areas of your life as finances, relationships, and creativity.

Feel the health of this energy flow. Is it strong or weak? Does it feel imbalanced or stifled? Take a few moments to better feel and tune in to the flow of this chakra.

Now tune in to the emotional energy of this chakra through clairsentience. What feelings emerge? Take your time feeling and naming the emotions as they surface.

You may want to ask the energy of this chakra to further communicate with you by asking more specific questions. Ask as many or as few of the following questions as seem important to you. Be alert and attentive to a slight increase in energy, a tingling feeling or low-grade buzzing sensation when you ask a question. This is a signal from the energy that there is more to explore in this area.

- "What emotions are keeping me from experiencing more financial abundance?"

- "Is there emotional energy stifling my ability to live a more creative life?"

- "What are my feelings and emotions surrounding sexual intimacy? Do I feel used? Do I use others?"

- "Is fear blocking me from pursuing a fulfilling career?"

- "How are my emotions—past, present, and future—affecting my health?"

Take your time with these questions. Ask them one at a time, then pause and be patient. Intuitive feelings will be persistent. You are likely to feel them or even think them. Be careful not to dismiss or deny what surfaces. The most damaging emotional energy is often buried and repressed because it is difficult to acknowledge.

In some cases you may receive clairvoyant images. You may see a memory of yourself that elicits long-forgotten feelings and emotions. It is possible that you will see and feel images of yourself that don't readily make sense. It might feel as if you are making them up. Again, remember that your imagination is the tool of your intuition. Allow whatever needs to surface to emerge in whatever way it needs to.

If uncomfortable or disempowering emotions surface, you can breathe and release them through the outbreath. Then inhale through the heart and send the energy of love and forgiveness into the second chakra.

Write down whatever you feel, sense, hear, and see.

The Solar Plexus Chakra

The third chakra is the solar plexus chakra. Located between the navel and the base of the sternum, its vibrational color is yellow. This is the center of our personal power, self-esteem, authentic self, and gut intuition. This chakra transmits life force energy into our personal power. It is the energy distribution center for integrating one's spirit into the personality self. When our personality or ego-self listens and acts on the direction and guidance from our inner spirit we experience authentic power. Fear dissipates and we outwardly express confidence and inner strength. The inner voice of our spirit leads us in ways that bring peace and contentment to our everyday lives. When our ego-self believes that it is its own source of power, we experience insecurity, vulnerability, stress, and anxiety. The world looks threatening and we believe that force and attack are necessary.

The intuitive information contained in this chakra has to do with our personal power, insecurities, stresses, fears, self-esteem, personality, ego, and our ability to listen to and trust our most basic instinctual and gut intuition. It governs the liver, middle spine, pancreas, gallbladder, colon, spleen, small intestine, stomach, and the digestive system.

Physical dysfunctions associated with a compromised third chakra are diabetes, pancreatitis, hepatitis, colon diseases, cirrhosis, digestive imbalances, intestinal tumors, eating disorders, hypoglycemia, chronic fatigue, hypertension, muscle spasms and disorders, adrenal fatigue, and arthritis.

Arthritis: The Prison of Fear

My phone session with Darlene began with her talking about herself. Unlike many of my sessions where people say very little, I had to jump in before she told me too much. It is always easier to intuitively tune in to another when you do not know a lot of their personal information.

Before I could stop her she told me, "I have been married for over thirty years. It has not always been easy. Jerry, my husband, is a good man, though. He works hard and likes his garden. We both like to garden. But I can't seem to bend over well enough to do much work in it these days. A friend of mine told me that maybe you could help me. The arthritis just keeps getting worse. I take so many medications, but I can't seem to tolerate them very well. My stomach has always been sensitive. Not that they seem to help too much anyway. The stiffness and pain just gets worse. I don't know what else to do."

I was finally able to stop her and said, "I need to intuitively tune in to your energy and see what I receive before you tell me too much."

When I tuned in to Darlene's body, I was surprised at the pain and soreness that she felt. She understated her discomfort. I saw raw red, dry, tight joints and inflammation throughout her body. I expressed what I saw to her and then began to explain the many images and feelings that I received, along with the physical information.

"I see an image of what I believe is your home. I feel that you have been living there for a long time. You spend a lot of time in it. Is this true?" I asked her.

"Oh, yes, we've been living here our entire marriage. Moved in when I was in my early twenties. I haven't seen much reason to leave."

"I see an image of you looking out the window. I feel stress and fear in your body. Your stomach feels tight. When I ask what you are worried about I see an image of a young woman. She has dark shoulder-length hair, an attractive woman. Is this your daughter?"

"That sounds like my daughter, Shelby. I also have a son, Jeffery," Darlene shared with me.

"I feel that you are worried about your daughter and your son. Your son lives close, but I get the impression that your daughter lives farther away. She feels busy. I'm not sure why you're worried about her. She feels content. I see children with her. These would be your grandchildren. They are beautiful children."

"I miss my daughter," Darlene chimed in. "I haven't seen her in a couple of years. Her husband got a job transfer. They live almost across the country. I do worry about her. Nothing specific. You know how life is, though. You never know what may be coming your way. Problems, accidents, illness—they take you by surprise."

"I'm not feeling that your daughter is in any danger or having any problems. She would love for you to visit her and see for yourself. Your fears seem to be limiting you from some of the good things in life."

"Oh, we couldn't drive all that way. I have never even been out of North Carolina. Never have flown in a plane and never will. Can't image how I will get out there to see her and the grandkids. I guess they will make it back here at some point," Darlene explained. "I am fine just where I am."

As I continued to tune in to Darlene's energy I could sense fear and feelings of powerlessness moving through her. It was causing the stiffness and tightness in her body. She seemed to lack any sense of personal power. I could see that she spent most of her time in the house, worrying about what might happen.

"You are safe. Your children are safe. Life wants you to know this. You can enjoy things more than you are. Get out into the sunshine. Imagine your fears and stress dissolving in the sunlight. Maybe have friends over or get involved with a hobby or social activity of some kind. I feel that your life force energy is stiff and this is making your body stiff and tight. As you relax, laugh, and enjoy simple pleasures more; your body will also loosen up. The arthritis does not have to debilitate you."

"I hear what you're saying. I would love to be getting out more, doing more. But, you know, it's hard. I don't have a driver's license, never got one. Don't know where I would begin. I have never been good at taking chances. Never been a strong person. Don't think I have it in me now to do anything but find comfort in this old house."

I continued to scan Darlene's body. We went through her medical problems and I offered her further insight into the concerns that she was troubled about. We talked about a few things like acupuncture and Reiki healing that would help. Unfortunately, she had let go of any personal sense of power to take care of herself a long time ago. Darlene's third chakra, like her arthritis, was tight and stiff. I offered her some suggestions for ways to stir up her inner power and find herself. When we hung up I sent a prayer for her to the angels.

Exercise: Claircognizance and the Third Chakra: Integrity and Power

This exercise will empower you to tune in to the energy of your third chakra and further develop the psychic skill of claircognizance.

Sit or lie down and breathe relaxing breaths. Focus your intuitive awareness between the navel and the sternum. Tune in to the circular vortex of energy of this area. Feel the flow of energy. Get an intuitive sense of the health of this chakra. Is it strong or weak? Does it if feel imbalanced or stifled? Take a few moments to better feel and tune in to the flow of this chakra.

The third chakra is your center of personal power and intuition. This is where gut feelings and intuitive knowing emerge from. Imagine that the energy of this chakra can communicate with you.

Ask this chakra to help you to tune in to your personal power and communicate to you through claircognizance. Remember to focus your awareness on the embedded mental intuitive energy of this chakra. It is easy to naturally direct your awareness in the thinking mind.

You may want to ask the energy of this chakra to further communicate with you by asking more specific questions. Again, be alert and attentive through vibrational sensitivity to a slight increase in energy, a tingling feeling, or low-grade buzzing sensation when you ask a question. This is a signal from the energy that there is more to explore in this area. Claircognizant energy information will surface as a gut knowing. This may be experienced as the awareness of undisputable certainty.

"Am I living my truth?"

"What are my beliefs about my intuition?"

"Can I trust myself?"

"If I allow myself to be powerful, what do I believe will happen?"

"What negative patterns of thinking are sabotaging me from experiencing what I most desire to manifest in my life?"

"How is the energy of my thoughts and patterns of thinking affecting my health?"

Take your time with these questions. Ask them one at a time, then pause and be patient. Intuitive thoughts will be persistent. Be careful not to dismiss or deny what surfaces. Sometimes repressed beliefs and thoughts are difficult to acknowledge.

In some cases you may receive clairvoyant images associated with the thoughts and beliefs that surface. Allow whatever needs to surface to emerge in whatever way it needs to. If negative and limited thoughts and beliefs surface, take note of them, then release them through deep relaxing breaths. Imagine breathing in positive energy that empowers you in every area of your life.

Write down whatever you feel, sense, hear, and see.

The Heart Chakra

The fourth chakra is the heart chakra. Located in the chest, this chakra vibrates to the color green and sometimes pink and is the energetic axis of love. The heart chakra absorbs all degrees and expressions of emotional energy along with the higher vibrations of divine love. Its function is to assist us in learning how to integrate the higher divine attributes of love—compassion, forgiveness, kindness—into our everyday lives and relationships. The ability to heal ourself and others and transmit cosmic healing energy into the world is centered in this area.

When we only know how to give love without receiving it, or if we expect to be loved but do not act in loving ways to others, this chakra becomes imbalanced. When we are fearful of opening our heart and expressing authentic emotions, this chakra becomes energetically blocked and shut down. This leads to a lack of vital source energy moving through the fourth chakra, the heart, and eventually the entire body. With a lack of healthy energy moving through the heart, illness and problems such as heart attacks, heart disease, strokes, and cardiovascular problems may result.

The intuitive information held in the fourth chakra has to do with our ability to transform our lower base ego emotions of anger, jealousy, fear, and conditional love with the energy of divine unconditional love. Our emotional fears, vulnerabilities, loneliness, our focus on materiality over emotional joy, and our relationship wounds, confusion, resentments, inability to forgive, and commitment issues are also stored in the heart chakra. This chakra reveals our ability to create balance in the love and care we give to others, with the love and care that we give to ourself.

This chakra is associated with the heart, circulatory system, blood, lungs, rib cage, diaphragm, thymus, breasts, esophagus, shoulders, arms, and hands. Common dysfunctions are heart disease, breast and lung cancer, lung disease, asthma, fluid in the lungs, shoulder, arm, and hand issues, carpal tunnel syndrome, immune disorders, circulatory problems, and issues with the thymus gland.

Anger in the Heart

Stan came in for a session with me on a cold wintery day. He had little to say and simply sat down on my couch and waited for me to begin.

As I tuned in to his energy I was drawn to his chest. His heart was struggling. It felt sluggish and at the same time I felt a tight band of energy restricting its normal rhythmic beating.

"I know this will be no surprise for you, I feel as if you have a heart condition. It feels as if you have been struggling with this for a while. But your condition is likely not improving," I told him.

"That's correct. My wife's friend suggested I come see you," Stan told me. "I have been to several different doctors. They all say the same thing. They tell me to take my medication, eat better, and exercise. Well, I have done all of those things. I don't smoke. I eat like a rabbit, and still I am not feeling any better. So I thought I would give someone like you a try. Anything helpful you can tell me?"

"I am happy to help you in any way that I can," I assured him. "Sometimes when we are not healing it's because there are nonphysical stresses and influences that affect our health."

"I'm not sure what you mean." Stan looked at me with a bit of apprehension.

"Let me take a look and see what I find. I'm not sure yet why this is important, but I see what looks like a wedding. It looks like a younger you getting married. You seem happy. Your bride seems happy. Yet, I get the feeling of frustration and anger. Despite the joy, there is also a feeling of loss," I shared with Stan.

"I'm not sure why you're getting this," he quickly told me. "That was one of the happiest days of my life and many years ago. I'm not sure I'm following you."

"There is also a man coming in from the other side. Is your father in spirit?" I asked.

"Are you asking me if my father is dead?"

"Yes, that's what I'm asking," I replied.

"He died several years back."

"He says that he is sorry. He is apologizing to you. I get the impression that this has something to do with the marriage. He says that you have a lovely wife," I explained to Stan.

Despite Stan's stoic demeanor, I could see him choking up.

"I am Jewish and I was brought up to follow the traditions and faith. My wife was not Jewish. She was very much a Christian. They never accepted her. We were married in a church, not a synagogue. It was difficult," he told me. "My father refused to come to the wedding."

"Are you still angry at your parents?" I asked Stan. "I feel a profound sense of anger and grief in your heart."

Stan took a moment then told me. "I cut them out of my life many years ago. Haven't seen or spoken to my father for over twenty years. He died of a heart attack a few years back. We never made our peace. He even cut me out of the family will."

"It's not too late," I encouraged Stan. "You can forgive him now. You can let go of the anger. It is affecting the health of your heart. The forgiveness is for you."

"I will try," Stan replied. "I know he didn't know any better. It probably contributed to his heart attack. I wish him the best. It's all down the river now."

EXERCISE: INTUITIVE HEALING AND THE FOURTH CHAKRA: THE HEART OF HEALING

As a medical intuitive you become a channel of hope and healing for yourself and for others. The energetic awareness moving through you, directing and guiding you, comes from a higher source. Its origin is in the divine vibration of love, wisdom, and cosmic unity. This energy can be experienced most directly through your heart chakra.

The following exercise will empower you to become more aware of the power of love and wisdom that is guiding, supporting, and healing you.

Sit or lie down and breathe long, deep breaths. Focus your awareness in your chest and tune in to the circular vortex of energy. Through vibrational sensitivity feel the energy of your fourth chakra. Is it open and flowing or does it feel as if the energy is restricted?

As you continue to breathe deep relaxing breaths, ask for higher vibration energy to move through the heart, cleansing and clearing this chakra. Continue to breathe and invoke high vibration energy. With the psychic skill of vibrational sensitivity feel the difference between your personal energy and the higher vibration energy that flows through you. This is the energy that heals and enlightens. You will know when your heart chakra is flowing with high vibration energy when you feel a tinging love and warmth move through you.

Receive this energy of love and warmth and breathe it in. Send it to any part of your body that is sore, tense, or tight. Take a few moments to feel this energy flow through you. Send this love and warmth to any emotional, mental, physical, or spiritual issue or concern. Take a few moments to allow this energy to go to wherever it is most needed. Keep breathing love and warm energy through the heart. Send this love and warmth to anyone who might need it. Keep breathing and ask this energy to then be sent out into the world. Feel the healing energy that flows through you.

Write down as best you can your experience of this love and healing energy.

The Throat Chakra

The fifth chakra is the throat chakra. It is located in the throat and vibrates to the color of sky blue. Empowering us to speak and express our truth, this chakra supports us in living and speaking with integrity and honesty. It assists us by funneling life force energy into our authentic self and then motivates us to express and share our truth with others. The ability to discern, make choices, and align our will with higher wisdom and guidance is also connected by this chakra.

We are always weighing what we want to share with others and the world and what we would rather suppress. When we express and share our authentic truth and individuality we flow within the powerful currents of life force energy. This is the way to health and well-being. What is stuck and repressed causes blockages and creates dysfunction. Expression creates movement. The spiritual challenge of this chakra is to release self-will and trust and allow the moment-to-moment emergence and expression of personal truth.

The intuitive information held in this chakra has to do with our attitudes, self-knowledge, confidence with self-expression, communication, and our fears of being judged and controlled by others and our environment.

This chakra is associated with the throat, teeth, gums, thyroid, trachea, neck vertebrae, esophagus, parathyroid, and hypothalamus. Health issues connected to this chakra are throat cancer, swollen glands, problems with the teeth and gums, laryngitis, chronic sore throat, thyroid issues, joint problems, and addictions.

Everyone Is Picking on Me

When I met Rita she was in pain. It was clear by the way she sat that moving her neck caused her discomfort. When I intuitively tuned in to this area of her body, I saw a couple of conflicting images. In one I saw what looked like Rita experiencing whiplash.

"I see you being shaken and jolted," I began. "I get the feeling that you have been in an accident within the past year. Actually ... it looks like you may have been involved in more than one."

"I was teaching my daughter how to drive. What a mistake that was," Rita interjected. "First time we got in the car, she hit a tree. We were not going too fast. My neck did get a bit of a jolt, though. But you're right, I did get into another accident a few years earlier. I got hit from behind while in heavy traffic. But I didn't think that one was too bad either. I've gone to physical therapy and even had acupuncture. This neck pain just will not go away."

"This doesn't feel like the only cause of your neck pain," I continued. "I get another image of you in what feels like your home. I get a lonely feeling. Almost as if you feel ostracized and disliked and you have no choice but to be alone. I feel a chronic tightness in your jaw. This feels to me like TMJ syndrome."

As I explained what I was intuitively receiving to Rita, she began to cry. I saw a look of fear in her eyes. I decided to give her a moment to process what I was receiving.

As I sat with Rita, I suddenly felt an angelic presence.

"There is an angel I just became aware of and she wants you to know that you are not alone, ever. She is with you. I get the message from her that it is time for you to be kinder to yourself. Even though it may seem that others are judging you, your worst critic is yourself. She says that the love and acceptance that you need must first come from within you. Then others will follow."

Rita had a skeptical look on her face. "I would like to think this is true. But I'm just not sure. I belonged to a book club for many years. I considered these people my friends. My opinions didn't seem to be accepted. Everyone just wanted to argue with me, it seemed. I got so afraid of sharing my thoughts, I just stopped. I don't say much now."

"It feels that holding back your true thoughts and opinions may be contributing to the tightness in your jaw and neck," I shared with Rita.

"I don't like being criticized. I feel like you may be judging me wrongly," Rita defensively told me.

I have learned over time that how I express what I intuitively tune in to is as important as what I receive. I knew that I was on dangerous ground with Rita. I did not want her to shut down on me and feel attacked. I took a moment and asked for help from the angelic realm. I knew that Rita needed a lot of support and healing.

"I'm sorry," I began. "I don't want to hurt you. I see another image of you as a young girl. You are sitting around a table. It looks like you're with your family. I'm getting a feeling of tension. I feel harshness and a critical attitude toward you. Maybe this is where some of these feelings stem from. Do you feel as if you were not always supported by your family?"

"That is an understatement if I ever heard one. My father was especially strict and even critical. We all had to sit around the dinner table and one at a time be asked questions and be drilled about our day at school. If the answer was not what my father wanted to hear, then he was not happy. I learned to say what he wanted to hear, then to just keep my mouth shut. Maybe this is affecting me now. It seems so long ago though," Rita told me.

"The part of you that felt judged and criticized when you were a child needs love and healing. Sometimes old issues resurface when we are strong enough and able to heal them. This might be the time for you to speak your truth, and love and support yourself—no matter what."

EXERCISE: CLAIRAUDIENCE AND
THE FIFTH CHAKRA: SPEAK YOUR TRUTH

This exercise will empower you to tune in to the energy of your fifth chakra and further develop the psychic skill of clairaudience. Clairaudience is the ability to hear energy information. Remember, this may manifest as either an inner hearing or an outer hearing. Often clairaudient communication is heard in what sounds like your own voice. Other times, it is distinctly different in tone and quality. Hearing clairaudient energy information will likely occur through inner hearing, and less frequently through outer hearing with our physical ears.

Sit or lie down and breathe relaxing breaths. Focus your intuitive awareness in your throat. Feel the circular current of energy of this area. Does the flow of energy feel open and expanded or imbalanced and tight? Get an intuitive sense of the health of this chakra. Is it strong or weak? Does it feel imbalanced or stifled? Take a few moments to better feel and tune in to the flow of this chakra.

The fifth chakra is the energetic center of communication and expression. It is embedded with both the positive and negative aspects of our ability to express our authentic self.

As you breathe and relax, send the inner message to your fifth chakra that you would like to communicate with it through clairaudience. Ask for guidance as to what is most important for you to express, to yourself and others, at this time. Then quietly listen. You may hear a still, soft voice, a more abrupt communication, or a repetitive inner message. These may sound like your own inner voice or an undistinguishable voice.

You may want to invite the energy of this chakra to further communicate with you by asking more specific questions. Again, be alert and attentive to a slight increase in energy, a tingling feeling, or a low-grade buzzing sensation when you ask a question. This is a signal from the energy that there is more to explore in this area.

Here are a few questions you may wish to explore:

- "Am I comfortable with communicating my thoughts and feeling to others?"

- "Do I keep quiet and go along with what others expect of me?"

- "What would I like others to know about me?"

- "What do I fear will happen if I am completely honest with myself and others?"

- "How is my reluctance to share my authentic self affecting my health?"

Continue to quietly listen to whatever surfaces. Let go of your expectations. Listen to anything else that the fifth chakra would like to communicate to you. Allow whatever needs to surface to emerge in whatever way it needs to.

Write down whatever you hear, see, feel, know, and sense.

The Third Eye Chakra

The sixth chakra is the brow chakra or the third eye chakra. It is located above and between the eyes and vibrates to the color indigo. Commonly referred to as the third eye, this chakra is the gateway for cosmic wisdom. It channels mind-energy consciousness and empowers us to become aware of possibilities, ideas, inspiration, and cosmic vision. Our thoughts, attitudes, beliefs, and judgments are meant to evolve. As we accept and contemplate higher truth and wisdom we are renewed and transformed. We become a spiritual being, empowered beyond the confines of physicality. When we stay stuck in our negative judgments, attitudes, and limited thinking and knowledge, we restrict the flow of life force energy. Our brain and mental functioning withers, shrinks, and short circuits.

It is through the sixth chakra that we become aware of spiritual reality. Clairvoyance, which is the ability to visually see energy information, emanates from the sixth and seventh chakras. This chakra opens our energy field and consciousness to the spirit realm. Within the sixth chakra is the doorway to see and commune with spiritual influences.

The inability to let go of addictive thought patterns and excessive mind chatter, along with the lack of self-evaluation, rejection of new ideas, and feelings of inadequacy impact the health of this chakra. When our thought consciousness does not evolve and accept higher truths and realities, we live in a very small and restrictive fear-based world. We recoil from the light of source energy and become overwhelmed with ego-based concerns and worry, and eventually become locked within the prison of our own self-judgments and limitations.

This chakra is associated with the brain, neurological system, eyes, ears, nose, and pituitary and pineal glands. Dysfunctions connected to the brow chakra are headaches, brain tumors, stroke, neurological disturbances, blindness, deafness, earaches, dyslexia, learning disabilities, seizures, Alzheimer's, mental illness and personality disorders, and sleep issues.

I Can't Hear You

Carl, an electrical engineer in his mid-fifties, came to see me on the recommendation of his acupuncturist. He was my last client on a long Saturday workday.

When I began to intuitively tune in to his sixth chakra I began to
hear a static buzzing. Initially thinking that it might be due to doing
too many readings, I stopped for a moment to take a deep breath. The
static cleared but began again as soon as I tuned into his sixth chakra. I
realized that this was not coming from me but from Carl.

"I hear a buzzy sound coming from your ears," I began. "Is this why
you're here? Are you experiencing a ringing of some kind in your ears?"

"Just one, I hear ringing in just one ear," Carl confirmed. "I have
been to so many doctors and specialists it would make your head turn.
No one knows what's going on. I have had so many tests— still nothing.
My acupuncturist thought maybe you could help."

As Carl was talking I continued to receive more information.

"This might seem off topic," I said. "But, you are very intuitive. You
have a large energy field, particularly around your sixth chakra. However, I feel suppression and tightness. Do you trust your intuition?"

"Well, it's not that I don't trust it. It's just that I don't have any need
to be intuitive. Don't want to complicate my life. I like keeping things
simple. If I can see it, touch it, or hear it, that's great. If not, I'd just as
well not pay it too much attention."

"Unfortunately, it is not really that easy." I tried to explain to Carl.
"It's kind of like saying, 'if I don't like what I see, I turn my eyes off.' Your
intuition is a normal part of you. It's as much of a functioning sense as
your five senses, and you know that you cannot ignore those."

"I guess you're right. But what does this have to do with the ringing in my ears?" Carl asked.

"I get the impression that when you were young, you were very
psychic and sensitive. I feel that you could intuitively see what others
could not see. Do you ever remember seeing spirits or deceased loved
ones when you were little?" I asked him.

"You are making me sweat a little," Carl said with a laugh. "Okay, I guess I did. I saw my grandfather after he died, walking around the house a few times. I will admit I also saw spirits in the woods near my house and sometimes in my house. To be honest, it scared me. I was afraid to tell anyone, so I just ignored it and willed myself to never see them."

"When we try to shut down and suppress our intuitive awareness and our psychic sight, it creates a buildup of energy pressure," I shared with Carl. "Because you are clairvoyant, which is the ability to visually see energy, your intuitive energy is centered in your head. This is where clairvoyance springs from. It's called the third eye. Over time this buildup of intuitive energy has created a blockage. What you hear is the reverberation of energy in your head. The doctors don't know what's causing the ringing in your ear, because they cannot detect it with their tests. This is why the hearing aid you tried didn't work either."

I continued the medical intuitive reading. Carl had a few other issues that needed to be addressed. Before he left we talked about a few ways that he could start to become more comfortable with his intuitive abilities. He seemed excited to re-explore this part of himself.

Exercise: Clairvoyance and the Sixth Chakra: See Your Way to Health

This exercise will empower you to tune in to the energy of your sixth chakra and further develop your ability to clairvoyantly see and perceive energy information. It is especially important that you use your imagination when you begin to develop clairvoyance. Your imagination will allow your intuition to make sense of the energy information you are receiving. The sixth chakra is your energy portal to higher truth and wisdom.

Sit or lie down and breathe long, deep breaths. Close your eyes and focus your attention in the brow area, between your eyes. Imagine a spiral flow of energy in this area. Remember to use your imagination. As you continue to breathe, imagine a portal of energy, like a doorway opening. As it opens, imagine that a funnel of energy expands in your line of vision and fills with color or colors. You may automatically begin to inwardly see color or colors or you may feel them or know what they are. You may just catch a short glimpse of these colors. Keep breathing and be patient.

Gently open your eyes and with soft, unfocused eyes, gaze into the center of your palm. Clairvoyance is not only seeing with human eyes, but with intuitive vision as well. What color or colors emanate from your palm?

Repeat this exercise. First close your eyes and imagine the portal of energy, then open your eyes and gaze into your hand with intuitive eyes. Keep repeating this process.

At some point you will be able to intuitively "see" energy.

You may want to ask the energy of this chakra to further communicate with you by asking more specific questions. Ask as many or few of these as seem important to you.

Be alert and attentive to a slight increase in energy, a tingling feeling, or low-grade buzzing sensation when you ask a question. This is a signal from the energy that there is more to explore in this area.

Breathe, close your eyes, and draw your awareness to the spiral of energy between your eyes.

Ask for an image to emerge that represents health and well-being.

Ask for an image of the food or foods that can be of most benefit to you at this time.

Ask to see an image of how the energy of this chakra is affecting your health.

See an image of yourself—joyful, happy, at peace, and healthy.

Record and write down all that you see and perceive.

The Crown Chakra

The seventh chakra is the crown chakra. It is located an inch or two above the head and vibrates to the color violet. The crown chakra absorbs cosmic life force energy and directs it through the aura and into the chakras and the meridians. States of pure spiritual illumination, acceptance of grace, and enlightenment emerge through this chakra. Concerned with our soul plan and its integration into our earth life, this chakra converts higher life force source energy, which exists outside of time, into three-dimensional workable phases. Keeping in sync with our soul's evolutionary agenda, this chakra is the bridge from timelessness to time. It empowers us to evolve through attracting and creating those opportunities that adhere to the lessons, challenges, and joys that we have come into the physical life to experience. This is the chakra that is responsible for disrupting the status quo and initiating change in our day-to-day lives. When we are not living our soul plan, the seventh chakra takes charge and sees to it that in one way or another we begin to pay attention. Events such as suddenly being fired from your workplace, confronting a life-threatening illness, divorce, and financial collapse are the calling card of the seventh chakra.

This chakra can also bring miracles and blessings into our lives. Your spirit is aware of everything that you do and experience. Every word, action, thought, and emotion is recorded and known. When we generate positive energy and listen and act on spiritual guidance, this chakra manifests goodness, love, and abundance in our lives.

Intuitive information contained in this chakra includes guidance from spirit guides, angels, and other divine beings. Past life influences, our soul plan, and life script can be accessed through this chakra. Stagnation and resistance to change, our unwillingness to surrender to our higher purpose, denial of spirituality, our inability to trust life, and selfishness create disharmony in this chakra. When we contribute to the common good, honor our spiritual self, become inspired, and act in faith, this chakra is filled with life force source energy.

Even though this chakra is not located in the physical body, it regulates and nurtures our overall physical, mental, emotional, and spiritual health. Physical dysfunctions associated with this chakra are depression, apathy, headaches, sensitivity to light, noise, allergies, multiple sclerosis, epilepsy, Parkinson's disease, senility, schizophrenia, paralysis, dizziness, dissociated states, panic disorders, and nervous system issues.

Panic Attacks

I talked to Lesley by phone. She had never before consulted with a psychic or medical intuitive and seemed very excited to begin.

"I never thought that I would be consulting someone like you," she told me. "But, I have learned never to say never. If you would have asked me a few years ago if I would ever talk to a psychic, I would have rolled over laughing."

I explained my process to her and we began. As soon as I tuned in to her energy field I felt an imbalance.

"As I scan your aura I feel a lot of energy in your higher chakras, particularly the seventh chakra. This is the area above your head. I get the impression that you have been actively participating in spiritual activity. You have been either meditating or spending time in contemplation," I told Lesley.

"Oh, that is true. How did you know this?" Lesley interrupted. "My yoga teacher was offering a class in meditation last year and I took it on a whim. I have been at it ever since. I love it. I am busy with my kids, but do everything that I can to make time every day to close my eyes and listen within."

As I moved deeper into Lesley's body I felt a powerful flow of energy move down her nervous system.

"It feels to me that you are in the midst of a transformation," I continued. "It feels powerful. I take it you are spending a lot of time in your spiritual pursuits."

"Like I said, I love it," Lesley answered.

The spiritual energy moving through Lesley was a bit overwhelming. The openness of her energy field was channeling in big waves of energy. It felt as if this was causing her nervous system to be on hyper alert.

I told her, "Sometimes when we spiritually open ourselves through meditation we can be flooded with energy. Think of high-vibration energy meeting denser physical energy. It can cause a bit of dissonance in our system. It can take a while to integrate this shifting from a purely physical material orientation to a more spiritual one. It is not only a shift in understanding but in energy as well."

"I'm not sure what you're talking about. I did go full blast into learning about spiritual things—meditating, chanting, and developing my intuition. But how would that not be good?" Lesley was clearly perplexed.

"I am getting an image of you as anxious and stressed. I can feel your system being overloaded. Do you ever feel panicky and hyper nervous while doing normal things like grocery shopping or driving the kids around?" I asked her.

"This started to happen to me a few months ago. I will be standing in line to buy milk and my heart races, my palms start to sweat, and I just want to run out of there as fast as I can. Sometimes when I take the kids to school this happens too. I thought meditation would help, so I have been doing more of it. Are you saying that meditation can actually make me nervous? This doesn't seem to make sense to me."

"The spiritual world is full of paradoxes. When we open ourselves to high-vibration energy it can simply take a while for our physical bodies to absorb the increase in energy. In past times it used to be that when we did intense spiritual work we had the protection of living in a monastery or on a quiet mountaintop. These days we go through these spiritual transformations in the midst of a busy and over-stimulated world. There is nothing wrong with you or your spiritual aspirations. It's just a matter of understanding the true nature of energy and learning how to take care of yourself and integrate better so that you will no longer experience these panic attacks."

I continued the medical intuitive reading and then shared a few grounding practices that I thought might help Lesley to integrate her spiritual and physical energy.

Exercise: Psychic Skills and
the Seventh Chakra: Receive Higher Guidance

This exercise will empower you to better communicate with helper spirits and higher vibrations of wisdom and love. The seventh chakra is your doorway to higher vibrational energy. It is also the chakra through which you can best feel and access the presence of your spirit helpers and angels. We have not yet discussed the role that spirit helpers and angels can play in your health and well-being. This information will come more fully in a later chapter. For now it is enough to become more aware of whatever loving, wise higher presence is supporting you in your efforts to develop medical intuition.

Sit or lie down and breathe relaxing breaths. Close your eyes and move your awareness to the space above your head. Tune in to the vortex of circular energy of the seventh chakra. Get a sense of the health of this chakra. Does it feel imbalanced, tight, loose, expanded, or contracted?

Breathe high vibration energy into this chakra. Move this energy through the body, letting go of any stress and tension. Continue to breathe down through the seventh chakra and feel this revitalizing energy move through you.

Ask for the presence of a spirit guide or angel that can guide you in the area of health and well-being. Be patient, and with the psychic skills of clairsentience, clairaudience, claircognizance, and clairvoyance become aware of whatever you feel, hear, know, and see. Let go of your expectations and remember to use your imagination. You do not need to receive a name, see your guides or angels, or know why a particular spirit helper is with you.

Some people will see a flash of color of deeper shades of magenta, gold, white, or turquoise. Others may see sparkles of energy and a translucent shimmering outline. It is also possible that you will see the image of an angel or spirit helper. You may also see symbols and images that may not make much sense.

Through clairsentience you may feel feelings of warmth, love, and comfort. You may also feel a warm hand on your shoulder, or a shiver of energy might move through your body.

Through claircognizance you may receive energy information about your spirit helpers or angels. They may also send you guidance about your health and well-being. This information may come to you through clairaudience. You might also hear soft whispers, a soothing melody, or the sound of gentle ringing bells. You might also hear the name of your angel or spirit helper.

Continue to breathe and receive as much intuitive energy information as possible.

Write down whatever you receive, even if you are not sure that it is coming to you from a guide or angel. Sometimes it takes some time for energy information to be fully understood.

Be sure to take your time with these exercises and repeat them as often as possible. With continued practice you will access deep levels of insight and important energy information. Not only will they enhance your intuitive knowing, you will also experience positive healing and new levels of health and wellness.

The next chapter is all about the important role that color plays in tuning in to and understanding the physical and subtle energy body.

12

THE VOICE OF ENERGY: COLOR AND VIBRATION

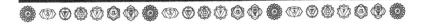

Color is visual energy. A universal language, color communicates meaning, form, and function. Our relationship with color begins at an early age when we learn the names of the different colors and then claim one as our favorite. Everything from religious items and spiritual principles to traffic laws and brand advertising can be identified by its symbolic coloring. Certain colors are connected to specific holidays, like red and green for Christmas and deep red and pink for Valentine's Day. We think of having a blue day as one that is sad or gloomy, and green often signifies envy and jealously. There are good reasons for our connection and utilization of color. Color is more than a descriptive and useful tool, it is alive with energy.

Isaac Newton performed the first scientific experiments concerning the origin of color. In his findings, published in 1672, he explored the colors of the rainbow and their relationship to light. He did this by setting up a prism in a sunlit window and observing the spreading out of color against a white wall. Newton realized that the colors red, orange, yellow, green, blue, indigo, and violet that he had observed resulted from bent or refracted rays of white light. He called this display of color a spectrum and concluded that white light contains all colors and blackness has none.

Through Newton's early experiments, we better understand that within white light there is an organized display of color. Through intuitive sight the true potency of color is revealed. Color is emitted from all living beings. It is vital life force energy and consciousness. Newton confirmed that the source of all color is white light. Through metaphysical and spiritual insight we know that white light contains the highest vibration of source energy and divine consciousness. It absorbs and transforms negativity and cannot be altered or contaminated. For the medical intuitive, white light and color contain useful energy information.

Vibration

The different hues of color are derived through its rate of vibration. The speed of light is measured at 186,000 miles/second. Albert Einstein studied light and determined that nothing could vibrate faster than the speed of light. Modern science, however, has since proven the existence of dimensions that are faster than the speed of light. "Light" is now known to be the dividing line between two different but related sets of existence. The material plane vibrates slower than the speed of light. The spiritual planes vibrate faster than the speed of light. Metaphysicians, poets, spiritual teachers, monks, and mystics have known this for centuries.

The physical body is comprised of molecules of light and vibrational frequency. Close your eyes for a moment and imagine your physical body as vibration and light. At some point while doing this, you may begin to feel that the different levels and speeds of vibration all work together as one network. Emotional energy vibrates to speeds just a bit faster than light and the mental planes are a bit faster than this. Your spiritual energy is even faster. The higher the vibration the closer you get to vital life force or white light source energy.

Each cell of your body vibrates at varying rates. Although you may feel as if you are one solid being, at your core level you are fluctuating levels of light vibration. Within every cell, vibrating molecules of memory, thought, and emotion are constantly created and dissolved. This cellular light activity is expressed as color. Through intuitive perception, the energy field or aura, the meridians, and the chakras are a colorful light show. For the medical intuitive, color and vibration are the messengers of mind, body, and spirit energy information. The vitality and luminosity of color communicates information about health, illness, and hidden or unconscious emotional, mental, and spiritual issues and imbalance. Color reveals your truth as it is the energetic container of your past and present consciousness, experiences, and beliefs.

The Seven Layers of the Aura

The aura contains seven layers of energy; each layer can be intuitively perceived as colorful vibrations of energy.

The first layer of the aura is associated with the root chakra. It is attuned to physical sensation, connectedness to the earth, and a sense of belonging. Its main color is identical to our primary core vibration color.

The second layer is associated with the sacral chakra. It is connected to emotional energy, creativity, and manifestation. The colors of this layer give insight into our range of emotions and our ability to interact with the material world. All colors of the rainbow can be seen in this layer. Bright, clear colors indicate health and vitality, while dark and clouded colors indicate depression, emotional wounds, or negative emotions.

The third layer is associated with the solar plexus chakra and our personal power, gut intuition, and self-esteem. This layer often has varying shades of yellow. Bright, clear colors indicate positivity and mental openness. Negative thoughts are connected to darker and cloudy colors. The third layer can often be perceived around the head as a yellowish halo.

The fourth layer is associated with the heart chakra and one's connectedness to cosmic and human love and relationships. With intuitive perception, this layer in a person with healthy spiritual energy can be perceived as a vibrant rainbow of colors.

The fifth layer is associated with the throat chakra and our will and ability to communicate and express our authentic self. Because this auric layer weaves in and around the other auric layers, its colors vary depending on one's authentic self and their predominant personality focus.

The sixth layer is associated with the third eye chakra. This layer is the interface between the spirit and human realm and inner sight and mental processing. Magenta and turquoise in this field indicate the presence of angels and spirit helpers. Many people intuitively perceive the color purple when developing their intuition. This layer of energy is our intuitive portal.

Lastly, the seventh layer is associated with the crown chakra. It contains our soul purpose, reveals the presence of divine helpers, and rules our spiritual and physical makeup. The presence of white and gold light in this chakra indicates a conscious connection with divine forces. The presence of dark shadowy energy can indicate a negative attachment.

Color and Vibration throughout the Aura

In addition to its core layer colors, the aura also contains a variety of other color-coded energy information. The location of certain colors, their shade, luminosity, texture, and structure all tell a story. Color in the aura or energy field provides energy information about your soul path, life lessons, your emotions, emotional wounds, your thoughts, and your physical health and well-being.

For the medical intuitive the energy vibration, shape, texture, luminosity, and presence of holes or other distortions in the aura are just as telling about the health and wellness of an individual as the color. A healthy aura is luminous and intact and contains clear, vibrant color. An aura with a distorted shape and empty spaces can signify fragmented energy. An energy field that is not unified and whole indicates imbalance in the mind, body, and spirit connection. A distorted and misshaped aura might also be caused by negative energy attachments or karmic present-life incarnation issues. At times a soul is pulled back to the earth by karma to complete soul lessons and evolve. When there is resistance to the karmic present-life incarnation, a part of the soul may resist and not come fully into the body. This eventually will result in emotional, mental, and physical dysfunction and illness. Karmic issues that negatively impact health are often best recognized through the quality of the aura.

Color in the Chakras and Meridians

Chakras as discussed in chapter 11 vibrate to specific colors. The first or root chakra vibrates to red. The second or sacral chakra to orange, the third or solar plexus chakra to yellow, the fourth or heart chakra to green, the fifth or throat chakra to blue, the sixth or brow chakra to indigo, and the seventh or crown chakra vibrates to the color of violet.

Like the seven layers of the aura each chakra also contains a variety of colors in addition to their primary color. For example, luminous green indicates healing energies. Magenta points to the presence of angels and angelic healing. Purple and gold can be a sign of divine beings. Quick flashes of translucent colors are associated with positive benevolent influences. Colors that are steady, consistent, and well-formed provide valuable insights and information about our thoughts, beliefs, emotions, and our health and state of being. Colors that are fleeting and fragmented may be harder to intuitively tune in to and may contain less substantial information.

Flow and Vibration

The name chakra is derived from the Sanskrit word meaning wheel, turning, and vortex. Chakras are spinning vortexes of energy vibration. They generally rotate in a clockwise direction, funneling life force energy into the body. However, chakras may rotate counterclockwise when detoxing and eliminating harmful energy. Either way, they should be spinning in a consistent rotation, neither too fast nor too slow.

Meridians vibrate and flow in a consistent pattern. For the most part meridians do not contain as much energy information as do the chakras and the energy field. However, if there is a physical illness, disease, or imbalance in the body you can detect this through the meridian's energetic flow.

Although I do not focus on the meridians in a medical intuition reading as much as I do the chakras and energy field, they can be especially helpful in providing detailed information about specific organs and bodily systems. Because meridians send life force energy into the body, they will alert you to specific issues. Once I intuit an imbalance in the body, I often follow the energy of the meridians to better know what organs and bodily functions are impaired. Muddy browns, gray, and murky or dull colors are signs that vital life force energy is restricted or blocked. Dark, hardened energy with lethargic or rapid vibration in the meridians indicates imbalance, illness, and/or disease.

The Meaning of Clear High Vibration Energy Colors

The color, shade, texture, and luminosity of color surrounding and within the subtle energy body are powerful indicators of our emotional, mental, spiritual, and physical health and well-being.

The following chart details the meaning and significance behind various colors in the mental, emotional, and spiritual layers of the subtle energy body.

Meaning of High Vibration Energy Colors	
Red	Power, life force energy, stability. A clear, bright red, ruby, or scarlet red indicate a passionate person who desires to bring about positive change in their life.
Pink	Love, harmony of earthly and spiritual love. A natural peacemaker, friend to those in need, close to children and animals.

Meaning of High Vibration Energy Colors (cont.)	
Orange	Creativity, ability to manifest, balance of spiritual and material consciousness. Clear orange indicates artistic ability and an individual who is open-minded and optimistic.
Yellow	Inspiration, ideas, intellect, logic, mind, and thoughts. Knowledge of all kinds, color of the communicator, and joyful personality. Might also indicate a performer or entertainer.
Green	Healing, protection, a loving heart, generosity, true humanitarian. A person with this aura color speaks from their heart and is trustworthy.
Blue	Communication, strength, confidence with self-expression, the color of the truth seeker, someone who has found the right path in life. Natural powers of leadership.
Purple	Conscious interaction with soul forces, spiritual vision, indicates a connection with wisdom, and a natural clairvoyant.
Gold	Harmony and balance, divine presence, perfection, immortality, the color of the visionary, the seer, one who can bring about widespread positive change.
Brown	Practical wisdom, grounding, a lover of nature and environmental issues, a nurturer, connected to Mother Earth.
Silver	Movement and transference of energy, gentle growth, feminine intuitive wisdom, may indicate pregnancy and conception.
Gray	A silver gray can indicate a fair, calming personality and a mediator.
Turquoise	Channel for divine forces into the physical plane, influencing, magnetism aides in healing, stimulating. The color of the wise healer, a poet, innovator, or artist.
White	Indicates divine source energy presence and healing. Many healers have concentrated funnels of white light in their energy field.

Detrimental Coloration

Colors that are low vibration—distorted, dull, shaded, dark, blotchy, murky, static, opaque, or excessive in quantity—indicate problems, imbalances, and/or the presence of negativity, toxicity, and attachments that can lead to illness and physical dysfunction.

	Dark, Muted, Shaded, or Clouded Colors
Red	Misuse or confusion with power, survival fears, egocentric, material minded, may be angry or overly sexual.
Orange	Imbalances in energy exchange between spiritual-physical realms, excessive drive, stifled creativity, apathy. Pale orange can indicate low self-esteem. A harsh orange can indicate eccentric behavior or an oversensitive ego.
Yellow	Overdependence on intellect and reasoning, judgments, limited thinking, critical, guilt, powerlessness, may indicate hyperactivity, resentment, and jealousy. A cloudy yellow indicates secrets and less-than-honest intentions.
Green	Excessive over-giving to exhaustion, codependence, looking to external world for satisfaction, loving to fulfill ego needs, jealousy, can indicate conflicting emotions and stress within current relationships.
Blue	Buildup of energy, stifled self-expression, lack of self-trust and confidence, depression, can indicate someone who likes to be in charge.
Purple	Ungrounded spiritual energy, distrust of intuition, inability to make decisions, can indicate a person who stays too long in fantasy, daydreams, and illusions, and a dark purple may indicate someone who feels alone.
Gold	Lack of self-awareness, over idealisms, can indicate a desire for material wealth at any cost, a preoccupation with worldly and ego power.
Pink	Unstable love, addiction to being in love, may be possessive with friends and family.

Dark, Muted, Shaded, or Clouded Colors (cont.)	
Silver	Hyperactivity, lack of centeredness, loss of energy, an individual who seeks excitement, physical stimulation.
Gray	Suggests depression, indecision, and stubbornness.
Brown	Focus in material consciousness, lack of spiritual awareness, can indicate over-indulgence and narrow vision of life.
Black	Depression or exhaustion, negativity, may also indicate an energy attachment.

Meaning of Subtle Energy Vibration and Flow in the Aura, Meridians, and Chakras

The vibration, movement, and flow of energy are as important as its color. Detecting energy flow is an essential sensory skill for the medical intuitive. When there is a high vibration and consistent flow of energy through the body, the cells, muscles, organs, and bodily systems are nurtured with vital life energy. Static, sluggish, and constricted color indicates imbalance, illness, and dysfunction in the body. The flow and vibration of energy can be detected by the texture and uniformity of color.

Meaning of Texture, Shape, and Vibration of Colors	
Color distortion or irregular shape	Willful battle between the ego and soul. Inability to evolve, obsessive personality. Too much or too little energy flow.
Holes in color, variegated, spotty	Loss of energy, lack of psychic protection, ungrounded, soul energy is not fully in body.
Hardened texture, static or dense	Energy block, prelude to manifestation of illness, disease in the physical body.
Color overlays	Control by another, manipulation of others, taking on another's energy as one's own.
Flashes of translucent color	Presence of positive divine energy, turquoise indicates spirit helpers, magenta the presence of angels, and flashes of gold and white divine presence.

Meaning of Colors Related to the Physical Body

When intuitively tuning in to the physical energy layer of the subtle body, color reveals the condition and wellness of the physical body. This color will be closer to the physical body, its vibration and flow will be slower and a bit denser than the color of the energy field.

Meaning of Colors in the Physical Layer of the Subtle Energy Body	
Bright red	The color of life force energy, health, and strength. Bright red is associated with healthy cells and the unhindered flow of blood and sexual potency.
Murky red	Can indicate recent injuries or surgeries, infections, blood problems, high blood pressure, fever, boils.
Physical association	Connected to the first chakra, blood, skeletal system, legs, feet, rectum, and coccygeal nerve plexus.
Clear orange	The color of healthy metabolism and immune system, regular pulse rate, fertility, hormonal balance.
Cloudy orange	May indicate problems with the reproduction system, menstrual pain, menopausal imbalance, impotence, allergies.
Physical association	Associated with the second or sacral chakra, the ovaries, large and small intestine, kidneys, spleen, and adrenal glands.
Bright yellow	Indicates healthy lymphatic and nervous system, good digestion, intelligence, ability to focus and concentrate.
Murky yellow	Can indicate tension, nervousness, exhaustion, digestive disorders, skin problems, rashes, arthritis, and rheumatism.
Physical association	Connected to the third chakra or the solar plexus chakra, rules the liver, digestive and nervous system, the joints, pancreas, gallbladder, colon, spleen, and small intestine.

Meaning of Colors in the Physical Layer of the Subtle Energy Body (cont.)	
Clear green	Indicates healing and positive regeneration taking place, healthy heart and respiratory system, stable blood pressure.
Murky green	Indicates colds, flu, viruses, chest or lung infections, bronchial problems. Can also indicate panic attacks.
Physical association	Connected to the fourth or heart chakra. Green rules the heart, respiratory system, lungs, thymus, breasts, esophagus, and shoulders, arms, and hands.
Clear blue	Balance and centeredness, stable blood pressure. Clear blue soothes pain and inflammation. Steel blue can indicate sharp pain, headaches, or migraines.
Murky blue	Can indicate depression, sluggishness, overactive thyroid, excess body weight, and lymphatic problems.
Physical association	Associated with the fifth or throat chakra, the throat, teeth, gums, thyroid, trachea, neck vertebrae, esophagus, parathyroid, and hypothalamus.
Clear purple	Harmony between the physical senses and the psychic senses. Mind, body, and spirit working as one. Presence of healing spirit helpers.
Murky purple	May indicate headaches, insomnia, nightmares, and eye, sinus, or ear infections. Cloudy murky purple may indicate memory loss and dementia.
Physical association	Associated with the sixth or third eye chakra. Purple rules the eyes, ears, head, scalp, and sinuses.
Clear pink	Balanced emotions, regular sleep patterns, relaxation, the presence of divine healing love.
Murky pink	Physical and emotional exhaustion, headaches, psychosomatic issues.
Physical association	Associated with the heart chakras, babies, and children.
Rich brown	Primal energy, physical strength.

Meaning of Colors in the Physical Layer of the Subtle Energy Body (cont.)	
Murky brown	Can indicate blockages in the chakras, toxins in the body, sluggish digestion, stress, overwork.
Black	Black spots may indicate tumors, severe blockage, or imbalance.
Clear gray	Can indicate stable moods, calm mind, strong physical constitution.
Murky gray	Depleted immune system, confusion, dementia, Alzheimer's.
Clear silver	Detoxing, releasing pain, healthy body fluids.
Murky silver	Water retention, sluggish lymphatic system, holding onto the past.
Clear gold	Powerful healing is taking place, vitality, long life, regeneration of body, mind, and spirit.
Murky gold	May indicate obsessions, compulsions, addictions.

MEDITATION: SUBTLE ENERGY COLOR

The ability to intuitively tune in to energy information through color and vibration is an important tool for the medical intuitive. The following meditation exercise will help you to better understand how the five psychic skills work together to provide useful energy information. It will also empower you to better tune in to the emotional, mental, and spiritual issues that influence your physical health.

In this meditation exercise you will use the psychic skill of vibrational sensitivity to tune in to the energy flow and vibration of the chakras and energy field. Then, using clairvoyance, you will visualize and inwardly perceive the color and/or colors of each chakra. The other psychic skills will provide additional energy information. Be patient with this process as you allow the energy color to further communicate energy information. Your imagination and intuition will work together to provide beneficial images and other intuitive sensations, thoughts, feelings, and guidance. In time this practice will feel more natural.

When tuning in to the energy of the chakras and the energy field remember to use vibrational sensitivity to become alert to energy that feels tingly, has a slight buzz, or lights up. This energy is trying to get your attention. Healthy, vital life force energy flows in a harmonious and balanced current. When there is an aberration in this flow, it will present itself as tingly, have a slight buzz, or light up. This indicates that the healthy flow of vital energy is being disrupted in some way.

You may want to have a recorder available or a pen and paper to take notes.

Close your eyes and begin to breathe long, deep relaxing breaths. Allow any thoughts and emotions to surface as you breathe. Take note of them and release them as you exhale. Continue to breathe and re-lease any tension or stress anywhere in the body. Continue breathing in this natural rhythm.

Focus your awareness in the first chakra. Using the psychic skill of vibrational sensitivity, imagine a red spiral of energy in the first chakra and tune in to this vibration. Continue to breathe as you draw your full attention to the energy flow of this area.

1. Breathe energy into this chakra and feel it expand. Imagine the energy of this chakra spreading out from your body about twelve inches in a circular orb.

2. Using clairvoyance tune in to any other color or colors within the center of the chakra. Slowly extend your awareness into the circular orb about twelve inches from the body. Take note of the location, size, and luminosity of any color or colors that are present. You may just catch a glimpse of color or light, or you may inwardly perceive many colors.

3. Scan the energy colors and notice if any light up, have a slight buzz, or feel tingly. Focus on one predominant color that gets your attention. If no colors light up, have a slight buzz, or feel tingly, move onto the next chakra or step.

4. As you focus on one of the colors, ask it to communicate with you. Breathe, relax, and receive energy information. With the psychic skills of clairvoyance, clairsentience, claircognizance, and clairaudience, pay attention to any images you receive, sensations you experience, anything you hear, any information that comes to you through a sense of knowing, and any feelings that surface.

5. Receive as much energy information as you can. Take note of it by writing it down or speaking into a recorder, then move onto the next chakra.

Move your awareness to the second chakra located a few inches below the navel. Imagine this as an orange spiral of energy. Continue with steps one through five.

Imagine a yellow spiral of energy in the third chakra and tune in to this vibration. Continue with steps one through five.

Take another long breath of white light energy and send it into the heart. Imagine a green spiral of energy in the fourth chakra and tune in to this vibration. Continue with steps one through five.

Imagine a blue spiral of energy in the fifth chakra and tune in to this vibration. Continue with steps one through five.

Take a deep breath and send it into the third eye area. Imagine a spiral of indigo energy in the sixth chakra and tune in to this vibration. Continue with steps one through five.

Breathe into the spiral of violet energy located a few inches above your head. Tune in to the vibration of the seventh chakra. Continue with steps one through five.

Take a long breath of white light energy and send it down through the spine. Imagine your chakras spinning in a humming high vibration. Send this vibration out through the chakras and into your energy field.

Continue to breathe in this way. Breathe white light down through the top of the head and send it down through the spine and then into the energy field. As you breathe draw your awareness about an arm's length away from the body. Tune in to the energy surrounding you. Get a sense of its parameters. Imagine that you have an inner intuitive antenna that can feel the oval- shaped energy that surrounds you. Breathe into this and feel its vibration, tune in to its luminosity, and notice any color or colors.

Breathe and imagine colorful pathways of energy running from the energy field back into the body. These meridian pathways are like ribbons of energy rippling through the body, sending vital life force energy through all of the organs and systems of the body. Feel the vibration of energy increase as you continue to breathe.

Release any negativity, stress, toxins, and anything that no longer serves you through the energy field. You are protected from any harmful or negative influences in this bubble of light energy. Imagine yourself as a colorful light show—vibrant, lucid, translucent, and alive with powerful streams of energy nurturing and strengthening you—mind, body, and spirit.

When you are ready open your eyes and write down your experiences. In this way you will ground and retain the awareness of yourself as healthy, vibrant energy.

Go through the color charts in this chapter to learn more about the colors that you perceived within your chakras and energy field. Based on the color, its location, and its luminosity or dullness, you can discover additional insights about yourself and your health and well-being.

Color and Vibration as a Healing Agent

All intuitive types can use the energy of color and vibration to promote healing in themselves and others. As you have learned, color is an important communicator of energy information. Color as vital life force energy can be used in sessions to bring balance, heal, and restore positivity. During medical intuitive sessions you can visualize healing color in areas where you detect illness, pain, or imbalances.

EXERCISE: COLOR HEALING

- Breathe relaxing breaths.

- Open your heart and imagine divine healing love moving through you.

- Become aware of the organ or bodily system, or emotional or mental issue that needs healing.

- Focus on this area.

- Imagine the area that needs healing overlaid with the color energy that is best suited for this issue.

- Imagine a spiral of high vibration energy in this same color.

- Imagine the spiral unfolding in the area where healing is needed. As the spiral opens and expands, healing energy and love is absorbed into the body, mind, and spirit.

- Repeat until you feel a decrease in vibration from the energy spiral.

- Close the area by imagining white light surrounding the area.

- Imagine white light moving through you, cleansing and clearing you.

Using Energy Color for Healing

White: Energy that vibrates to the color white is clear, translucent source energy. It is divine light. White is the perfect color, for it is all color. It is the color of goodness, purity, perfection, perfect balance, and harmony. When used for healing, white light protects, heals, enlightens, detoxifies, cleanses, clears, uplifts, repairs, eases pain, restores, transforms negativity into positivity, and signals the entry of divine forces and beings. Direct white light to any part of body, problem, or issue that needs healing.

Red: Red is connected to the first chakra, the root chakra. It stimulates, brings warmth and energy, and is good for fatigue and cold. Red supports blood circulation, strengthens the blood and the heart, and it heightens low blood sugar. Use for overall invigoration of the organs; it stimulates the five senses and the nervous system, and promotes healing of chronic infections and wounds.

Orange: Connected to the second or sacral chakra. Orange brings warmth and stimulates joy, optimism, and creative thinking. Increases appetite, relieves cramps, spasms, and gas, and builds bones. Use for perimenopause balance and premenstrual pain.

Yellow: Connected to the third chakra. Stimulates higher thoughts, increases confidence and cheerfulness; yellow strengthens the nerves and the mind. Increases metabolism, aids the lymphatic, granular, and digestive systems. Use for conditions of the liver, intestines, and stomach.

Green: Connected to the fourth or heart chakra. Powerful healing color; green aids the entire body and can be used for almost any condition in need of healing—cools, soothes, and balances. It is both energizing and harmonizing. Cleans and purifies germs and bacteria, rejuvenates the heart, increases immunity. Use green for the lungs, diabetes, ulcers, and joint problems. Calms and cools fever, high blood pressure, and skin irritation. Soothes and calms anger, aggression, or nervous conditions.

Blue: Connected to the fifth or throat chakra. Cools and relaxes the mind and body. Reduces fever, irritation, and pain; use for treating burns, high blood pressure, and inflammation; can be used for sleeplessness, phobia, endocrine imbalances, and to calm the pituitary and pineal glands.

Indigo: Purifies the bloodstream and circulatory system, and strengthens the endocrine system. Detoxifying; stimulates the spleen and immune system, decreases pain, and aids in healing addictions, delusion, and melancholy.

Brown: Grounding, protection of pets, heals animals, brings material stability, and increases decisiveness and focus.

Magenta: Use magenta to attract healing angels. Magenta is especially helpful for people who are complacent and need to activate their own healing powers.

Turquoise: Also a color that signifies angelic help and the presence of spirit guides. Use to ease mental and emotional stress, panic, and anger, and bring a sense of calm and serenity to highly tense situations and dispositions.

Pink: Softens emotional wounds, brings comfort to the grieving, eases tension and stress.

Use one or more color vibration at a time. Allow your intuition to lead you as to what colors will be the most beneficial. Despite the energy that each color vibrates to, color combinations can create new and useful healing energies.

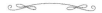

Perceiving self as energy, color, vibration, and consciousness opens up new perceptions and possibilities for healing, self-awareness, and empowerment. Practice the exercises in this section as much as possible and become familiar with the meaning of color. As your mind accepts new ways to observe and make use of your intuitive senses the process will become easier and more natural.

The next section brings together all that you have been learning about energy, color, vibration, accessing energy information, and the psychic skills. You will learn and practice how to better tune in to your health and how to conduct a medical intuitive session with another.

Section 4

MRI Scan: The Medical Reading & Intuitive Scan

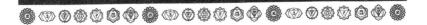

13

THE INTUITIVE
SELF-SCAN PROCESS

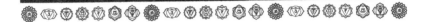

Harness the power of your intuition to access important health energy information when you most need it. Although your intuition is always communicating to you, there will be times when you may have a specific health question or want a more candid and penetrating observation of your physical body.

The two exercises in this chapter access medical intuitive energy information in different ways and for different purposes. The intuitive type exercise will empower you to tune in to a specific area of concern or question. The intuitive body scan provides you with a comprehensive overview and a detailed examination of your physical health and the mental, emotional, and spiritual influences affecting it.

MEDITATION: INTUITIVE SELF-SCAN CLEARING

Intuitively tuning in to your own health and well-being involves a slightly different process and experience than tuning in to the health of others. It is not always easy to let go of our personal bias and preconceived thoughts and beliefs. To tune in to and receive clear and accurate intuitive energy information it is necessary to adopt an open beginner's heart and mind.

You are energy and consciousness. Allow the wise inner voice of your spirit to intuitively guide you. Pure universal life force energy flows into your energy field, chakras, and into your physical body. This high-frequency vibration feeds, nourishes, and sustains your organs and bodily systems. Your thoughts, emotions, experiences, and memories also pull from this force field of energy. Negative and limited beliefs and thoughts, fear, anger, repressed grief, and resentment move you out of alignment with this pure life force energy. It robs your body of the energy that it needs to maintain good health.

The emanations of this energy are constantly sending you intuitive messages about your health and well-being. We have an inner set point to health. The miniscule molecules that comprise your being vibrate toward the light of the divine. Negative thoughts, emotions, memories, fears, and experiences lower your vibration. Every fiber of your being calls out to you to release and heal whatever it is that stands in the way of absorbing and becoming one with the pure energy of light. Intuit from the center of this perception and pure awareness.

Intuitive Type Messages

As you become more aware of your intuitive type, your subtle energy body, and the psychic skills, you can use your intuition for good health and healing on a daily basis. You are likely already receiving an increase in intuitive health messages. These messages may be understated. So much so that you might disregard and tune them out. Intuitive awareness does not always arrive in a mysterious and earth-shattering way. Receiving energy information about your personal health can be quite simple.

The intuitive messages that you receive will most likely surface through your predominant intuitive type.

An emotional medical intuitive often experiences health messages through either positive, uplifting feelings or through feelings of anxiousness or foreboding fear. Whatever promotes feelings of love and inner peace increases the flow of positive life force energy through your mind, body, and spirit. In the same way behaviors, habits, and activities that leave you feeling frustrated, melancholy, or unsettled are likely not good for your physical health. Long-term repressed feelings such as grief, loss, and fear, and negative feelings such as anger and resentment create energy blocks in your subtle body and eventually surface as illness, chronic pain, or disease in the physical body. Intuitively uncovering negative feelings and allowing old wounds to surface discharges the toxicity of these emotions and promotes healing and an improved sense of well-being.

Prior to the onset of an illness or disease, emotional intuitives may feel uneasy, restless, and hyper, or depressed and lethargic. We all feel this way from time to time, so if these kinds of feelings persist, listen within to your intuition for more insight and guidance.

For the mental intuitive, messages often surface through incessant thoughts and quick knowing. Unlike the emotional intuitive, these messages are not emotional in nature. They tend to be quiet, persistant, short, and to the point. Intuitive messages that warn or alert of a health condition can become repetitive. These thoughts can be vague, such as, "*something is wrong,*" or "*go to the doctor.*" The messages can also be more direct, such as, "*my blood sugar is off,*" or "*it's time to get a mammogram.*"

More attuned to physical sensations and body messages, the physical intuitive receives intuitive insight in a more physical way. They may feel an uncomfortable twitch, a subtle physical sensitivity, or a subtle pain in a part of their body. Yet, these slight sensations seem to have no known source, as they surface before any confirming sign of a health issue or problem. Some physical intuitives may seem to their friends and families to be hypochondriacs. They may talk about a health problem or concern without showing any physical symptoms. However, the difference between an intuitive message and a neurotic fear is that an intuitive message, when listened to, also provides practical and healing guidance.

A spiritual intuitive may receive health messages through feelings of being led by an invisible force. Their dreams may reveal an unknown health issue and they are more aware than the other types when a loved one on the other side or an angel tries to alert or warn them of a potential health problem. Like mental intuitives they often have a spontaneous awareness and knowing of a physical problem or imbalance. However, they do not receive the energy information through a mental thought but more through a flash of insight. Spiritual intuitives are also more sensitive to shifts and changes in their energy level. They may feel a lack of vitality or an inner sense of energy stagnation and intuit that this is connected to a physical issue.

EXERCISE: INTUITIVE TYPE HEALTH QUESTION

However your intuition naturally surfaces, you can harness the random, spontaneous, and often confusing intuitive messages into practical information. Using your intuitive type and the medical intuitive skills, you can invoke energy health information when you most need it. The more you listen and act on what you receive, the stronger your intuition becomes.

This meditation exercise will help you to better tune in to personal health energy information and intuit through all of the different intuitive types. Use it when you suspect that your intuition is trying to give you a health-related message or if you desire specific information about your health.

Before you begin this exercise, think of a health-related question. This question can be about any area of your health and well-being. You can ask for guidance about your mental, emotional, or spiritual health, but keep it simple and specific.

It is best to not ask too broad of a question like: "*Is there anything that I need to know about my health?*"

Instead a more simple and direct question would be: "*How can I improve my metabolism?*" Or "*Are my feelings of uneasiness and anxiousness related to a potential health problem?*"

- Write down one specific question. Then take a few minutes to write down any thoughts or feelings about this question. What do you think your intuition will tell you? Write it down. Thinking and writing down your thoughts before you begin will help to clear your mind of preconceived expectations. It will be easier to receive and trust your intuitive impulses.

- Begin by closing your eyes. Slowly inhale and move the energy of the breath through the body. Exhale any stress and tension through the outbreath. Continue to breathe and relax and exhale any stress or tension through the outbreath.

- As you continue to breathe imagine your mind and heart opening. Continue to breathe deep cleansing breaths, releasing any tension and stress through the exhale.

- Ask your question either aloud or silently within. Repeat it a few times. Breathe and listen and ask for an image to emerge that represents your question. Use your imagination. You do not need to understand the image. Just become aware of it. This is the intuitive skill of clairvoyance.

- When you feel as if you have received all you can from the image at this time, inhale and exhale a deep breath. Take a few moments to breathe, repeat the question, and tune in to whatever emotions surface. This is the intuitive skill of clairsentience.

- When you feel as if you have received all of the emotional energy that you can at this time, inhale and exhale a deep breath. Ask your question and pay attention to your thoughts. Listen within for the still, small voice. You may hear an inner message that feels as if it is your thoughts. Pay attention to whatever surfaces. This is claircognizance.

- When you feel as if you have received a knowing or an inner message, inhale and exhale a deep breath. Ask your question and tune in to your body. Become aware of any physical sensations and pay special attention to your gut knowing. For this exercise you do not have to understand everything you experience. Simply take note of whatever you feel and receive. Tuning in to bodily sensations is another form of clairsentience.

- When you feel as if you have received an intuitive message through your body, inhale and exhale a deep breath. Tune in to the flow of energy through your body. This is vibrational sensitivity. If you feel any tension, stress, stagnant or erratic energy, imagine this energy to be color. You may perceive, feel, sense, or simply know the color or colors. What is the texture and color of this energy? What is the color telling you? Use the color charts to better understand the meaning of these colors.

- If you have received any feelings, thoughts, bodily sensations, or images that you do not understand, focus on them one at a time. Dialogue and communicate with whatever you receive. Ask simple questions and then patiently breathe and listen.

- Write down what you experience as it may fade as you come into normal consciousness. When you have received all that you can at this time, send gratitude and love to the spirit realm.

- Remember to keep your questions concise and direct. The more often you consciously listen within, the more you will intuitively receive and understand.

Self-Scan

In a medical intuitive self-scan you have the opportunity to use all that you have previously learned and practiced to conduct a complete health scan for yourself. In a medical intuitive session the complete body, mind, and spirit are acknowledged and considered. Not only will you be scanning the physical body for disease, dysfunction, pain, and imbalance, you will always look into how emotional, mental, and spiritual energy influences the overall experience of good health and well-being.

Preparation for Intuitive Body Scan

An intuitive body scan is the most direct way to tune in to physical health. Not only will a comprehensive intuitive scan reveal physical illness, imbalances, and disease, it will also uncover the emotional, mental, and spiritual issues underlying them. Be well rested and set aside at least an hour to complete it.

Before you begin the scan find a quiet place where you will not be disturbed. Have a pen and paper or a tape recorder close by that you can record your intuitive impressions as you receive them.

Prayer

You may want to begin a self-scan with a prayer to invoke and invite the highest love, wisdom, and guidance to be a part of your session. When you ask for the presence of your spirit helpers, angels, and the highest vibration of light, you are supported by powerful spiritual assistance. You call your spirit forward and allow yourself to be guided.

You might want to use something like this:

Mother, Father, God (divine spirit, presence, universal love, etc.—whatever you are comfortable with)

I ask for the white light of your love and protection. I also ask for my angels, spirit helpers, loved ones on the other side, and my highest self to come close. Provide me with insight, guidance, wisdom, and healing energy for my emotional, mental, spiritual, and physical health and well-being.

Meditation: Cleansing

After you invoke spiritual help through a prayer, a cleansing meditation will help you to open to intuitive guidance.

Find a comfortable, quiet space where you will not be disturbed. You may want to have a voice recorder or pen and paper close to record what you intuitively receive.

Begin by closing your eyes. Slowly inhale and move the energy of the breath through the body. Exhale any stress and tension through the outbreath. Continue to breathe and relax.

Breathe in white light energy and allow it to circulate through your body, loosening and relaxing any stress and tension. Then exhale through the heart. Feel your heart begin to open. Release any negativity, old wounds, and hurts through the outbreath. Bathe your heart in the divine breath.

As you continue to breathe in white light, imagine your mind opening. Feel your consciousness expand as your mind merges with the divine mind. Feel the presence of love as soft energy filling your mind, heart, body, and soul. Continue to breathe in this energy. Rest, open, and allow love to fill you.

When you are ready, send warm thoughts of love and gratitude to the spirit realm. Ask to be divinely guided in tuning into your health.

The Scanning Process

A body scan involves moving your intuitive awareness through your body one section at a time—creating images for each area and communicating with the energy to receive health energy information. Imagine seeing the area on a blank screen. During a self-scan if may feel awkward to intuit your own energy and physical self in this way. You may feel drawn into your energy and you may want to use your thinking mind instead of your intuition. Unlike scanning others, in a self-scan it is necessary to balance both an objective and personal perspective.

How Energy Gets Your Attention

As in previous exercises remember that if an image of your body lights up, tingles, has a buzzing vibration, or if you feel a hardness or inertia in the energy flow, this is an indication that there is a dysfunction or problem. In this case ask to see another image of the problem area. Once you perceive an image of the problem area, ask the following questions one at a time. The energy will respond by providing you with energy information through another image. If you do not understand the image, ask for another image, thought, or emotional insight to clarify. Continue to communicate with the energy.

Expect the energy of an area to communicate to you through images. Allow your imagination and intuition to work together to create clairvoyant images of the area that you are intuitively tuning in to. Remember you may intuitively feel, know, or sense an image, you do not have to visually see it.

The Questions

Questions to ask the energy images:

- *How is this energy manifesting in my body?*

- *If this energy had a voice what would it be saying?*

- *What is the emotional energy of this image?*

- *What is the mental thought energy or beliefs and attitudes associated with this area?*

- *What message does my spirit have for me in connection to this issue?*

Not all of these questions will be answered. The ones that are important for the area of the body you are scanning will have more energy. This may feel like a tingle or you may see a sparkle of light. In time you will be better able to discern the presence of important energy information.

Be Patient with the Process and with Yourself

During a scan you may initially receive little intuitive energy information. Or you may receive quite a bit and feel overwhelmed by it.

The energy information that you receive may feel fuzzy, confusing, and you may not be able to decipher what you receive. Do not panic. This is normal. Instead of becoming stressed by this, pat yourself on the back for your ability to receive intuitive energy. You do not need to figure it all out. Just receiving energy information says that your intuition is working.

Become an Observer

Assume several different points of awareness. Part of you is the intuitive observing. You are just taking in energy information. You do not need to understand everything you receive. Just receive. Another part of you will be anxious and stressed and wondering if you are doing this correctly. Don't give these concerns too much attention. Simply acknowledge your fears and let them go. Another part of you may become triggered by the questions that you are asking. You may acutely feel the emotions that surface. Memories that unexpectedly emerge might provoke surprising revelations and insights. New awareness about your physical body, your health, your beliefs, and negative attitudes may make you uncomfortable and uneasy. As much as possible allow yourself to be present to the emotions, thoughts, and insights that surface, and at the same time stay as connected as possible to your observer self.

Take Your Time

You can do part of the scan and stop. You do not have to complete it all in one session. It might be a lot to take in and process at one time. If this is the case, end the session and continue where you left off when you feel more rested and ready.

Exercise: Self-Scan

Use your psychic skills of clairvoyance, clairsentience, clairaudience, claircognizance, and vibrational sensitivity to tune in to the energy information that you are given. Pay attention to the luminosity, brightness, or muted shades of the colors. Refer to the color charts for help in deciphering their meaning and significance.

Write down or speak into a recorder whatever information you receive. Do not try to fully understand or diagnose an issue at this time. If you hear a medical term that you do not understand, write it down and look it up in a medical dictionary later. Once you have received all that you can in this area, move on to the next. You do not need to fully understand what you are receiving to continue. Quite often you will gain more insight as you continue with the intuitive scan.

If an image does not light up and the energy flows smoothly, move onto the next area.

I begin medical intuitive readings in the seventh chakra, which is above the head. This reinforces the presence of spiritual energy and provides an overview of the flow of vital life force energy through the body. You will scan your body section by section.

After the cleansing meditation you can immediately begin the intuitive scan.

- Focus your awareness in the seventh chakra. This is slightly above your head. Breathe a long deep breath and relax. Imagine an energy spiral above your head. Breathe into it. Ask to view this energy spiral on a blank screen. Notice its colors, texture, and feel the vibrational flow of energy move through it. Once you have viewed an image of this spiral ask for the spiral to spread out to the width of your energy field. Imagine this spiral of energy as four sections: front, right side, back, and left side.

1. Begin to scan section by section in a clockwise motion. Ask for an image of each section one at a time. If the area lights up, has a slight buzz, or if you feel an inertia or hardness in the energy flow, ask to see an image of the problem area.

2. Questions to ask the image:

- *How is this energy manifesting in my body?*

- *If this energy had a voice what would it be saying?*

- *What is the emotional energy of this image?*

- *What is the mental thought energy or beliefs and attitudes associated with this area?*

- *What is the spiritual message connected to this issue or area?*

3. Not all of the questions will be answered. The ones that are important for the area of the body that you are scanning will have more energy. This may feel like a tingle or you may see a sparkle of light. Write down or record what you receive. You will know that you have sufficiently and thoroughly received all of the information when the area that you are viewing no longer lights up or flashes energy. It will emit a calm, toned-down energy that no longer is trying to get your attention. When this happens move onto the next section.

- Once you have completed all four sections of the expanded seventh chakra energy spiral, you will now scan the energy field. Starting at the seventh chakra above the head, imagine the energy field completely surrounding your body. Segment the energy field into four sections: front, right side, back, and left side. Scan one section at a time in a vertical manner, asking for an image of each section. If a section lights up, flashes energy, or if you feel inertia or hardened energy ask to see an image of the problem area and then proceed with steps one through three. Write down or record what you receive. When a section no longer lights up, move on to the next section.

- When you have completed all four sections of the energy field, move your awareness to the sixth chakra. Become aware of a spiral of energy in the center of your head. Ask the energy to encompass the entire head and expand a few inches outside of the head. Segment the energy field into four sections—the brain, the sinus and face, the eyes and nose, and then the ears and teeth. Scan one section at a time, asking for an image of each section. If a section lights up, tingles, or if you feel inertia or hardened energy, ask to see an image of the problem area and then proceed with steps one through three. Write down or record what you receive. When a section no longer lights up, move on to the next section.

- When you have completed scanning the sixth chakra, move your awareness to the fifth chakra, the throat area. Ask the energy to expand to encompass the throat and shoulder area. Segment this area into the neck, the throat, the shoulders, and then the arms and hands. If a section lights up, flashes energy, or if you feel inertia or hardened energy ask to see an image of the problem area and then proceed with steps one through three. Write down or record what you receive. When a section no longer lights up move onto the next section.

- Once you have scanned this area move your awareness to the fourth chakra, the chest area. Feel the energy spiral of the fourth chakra. Ask for this energy to expand and include the heart and lung area. Expand this energy a few inches outside of the body. Divide the chest area into the heart, the bronchial tubes, the lungs, and the breasts. Ask for an image to appear on the blank screen that represents the energy of each area one at a time. If an image lights up, or feels hardened and inert, ask for an image that represents the problem. Continue with steps one through three. When you have received as much information as possible the image will fade.

- When you have completed scanning your chest area move your awareness to your solar plexus. Imagine an energy spiral within your abdomen. Expand this spiral to encompass the entire area extending about two inches outside of the body. Separate this area into the stomach, the gallbladder on the right side, the liver on the right side, the spleen on the left side, and then the pancreas on the left side. Scan each section one at a time. Again, as in previous sections, ask for an image of each section, if it lights up, or feels hardened or inert, ask for an image of the problem and continue with steps one through three.

- Once you have completed the solar plexus scan move your awareness to a few inches below the navel. Imagine a spiral of energy within the body and ask this energy spiral to expand to encompass the entire area, including a few inches outside of the body. Separate this area into the colon, which lies across the stomach; if you are a woman scan the ovaries on the right and left side and the uterus, if you are a man scan the prostate; then scan the bladder low center. Scan each section one at a time. Again, as in previous sections, ask for an image of each section; if it lights up, or feels hardened or inert, ask for an image of the problem and continue with steps one through three.

- When you have completed scanning this section, move your awareness to the lower part of the body. Imagine a spiral of energy within the body and ask for this spiral to expand to encompass the entire lower part of the body. Separate this area into the spine, the right and left kidney, the lower colon, and the legs and feet. Scan each section one at a time. Ask for an image of each section, if it lights up, tingles, or feel hardened or inert, ask for an image of the problem and continue with steps one through three.

- When you have completed scanning this section, move your awareness to a spot a few inches below your pubic bone.

Intend to scan the endocrine system. Ask for an image of each gland. Begin with the ovaries if you are a woman and the testes if you are a man. When this scan is complete move your intuitive awareness to the adrenals, then the thymus, thyroid, pituitary, and then the pineal. Ask for an image that includes the energy of the glands flowing in unison. Scan this image. If this image does not light up or draw your attention in any way you have completed this area. If it does light up, ask for an image that represents this area and continue with steps one through three to further understand the problem.

- Move your attention down to the soles of your feet. Imagine a spiral of energy and ask this energy to expand through the entire body. Ask to view one at a time the lymphatic system, the circulatory system, the nervous system, and the skeletal system. Ask for an image of each section. If an area lights up, tingles, or feels hardened or inert, ask for additional information and continue with steps one through three. Scan each section in this way.

- When you have completed this scan, imagine a spiral of energy at the top of your head. Ask for the presence of divine healing energy to enter this energy spiral. Ask that this energy spiral of white light healing energy move through your entire body and energy field. Breathe, take your time, and allow this energy to move through you, healing and cleansing and revitalizing your entire self—mind, body, and spirit.

- When you have completed this energy healing, imagine a white light orb of energy completely surrounding you. This orb of energy will continue to heal and protect you from external negative influences.

- If you have detected any illness, dysfunction, disease, or simply feel uncomfortable with what you have intuited, follow up with conventional and alternative medical professional help. Heal whatever emotional wounds you have uncovered, forgive those toward whom you hold resentment and anger, transform your limited and negative attitudes and beliefs, and continue to let go of what no longer serves your highest degree of health and well-being.

Self-scans provide us with a deep and complete intuitive look into our health and well-being. Take your time with the scan. Do as much as you can do in one session, record what you receive, and then continue with the scan when you feel rested and rejuvenated. Self-scans can provide an enlightening and fascinating glimpse into ourselves. Enjoy the process.

What to Expect and How to Interpret It

With both of these exercises and with the intuitive scan for others in the next chapter, you are likely to receive different varieties of intuitive messages, sensations, feelings, images, colors, and vibrational stimulation. It is not always easy to decipher and interpret everything that you receive.

Here are some general guidelines to help you better understand the energy information that you intuit during these exercises, when performing a medical intuitive scan for another, and with intuitive impressions in general.

Refer to Color, Chakra, and Aura Information

Pay attention to the colors that you intuit and the physical area from where you are receiving intuitive information. Write down or record your impressions, and when you have completed the intuitive process, review the inherent meaning within the colors and the areas from where you have received energy information.

The seven chakras and layers of the energy field contain an immense wealth of physical, emotional, mental, and spiritual energy material. The energy of these areas can reveal and disclose significant and important issues, influences, and patterns of thought, emotions, beliefs, and choices that are at the root of illness, pain, and disease. Re-read the sections in the past chapters that have to do with the chakra areas from where you have intuited energy information and the colors that you have received. Ponder and examine it for additional clues and insights to assist in accurate interpretation.

Trust Your Interpretation

Trust your initial impressions. To understand the meaning behind intuitive impressions, it is necessary to draw upon your inner knowing. Some symbols, colors, numbers, and images have universal interpretations. While it can be helpful to know these common definitions, no one can interpret what you receive better than you can. Even if you do not realize it, you have a personal inner code of understanding that you have worked with all your life. As you develop your own intuitive abilities, you will learn to trust and rely upon that code.

Use your intuition to interpret. Accurate intuitive interpretation involves both the left and right brain. Allow your thinking mind to suggest an interpretation. Use your right (intuitive) brain to confirm, and get a sense of what feels correct.

Do not feel pushed to figure out and understand everything.

Give yourself time to correctly interpret and understand everything that you receive. Let go of the expectation that you will quickly understand all of the energy information that you intuit. Document what you intuitively experience and don't feel rushed to interpret it. It is enough to elicit energy information. You do not have to know what to do with it at the time of the scan.

Simply communicating with your body, caring enough to love and attend to you, activates healing.

Intuited Thoughts

Intuitive thoughts are persistent and usually steady in vibration. They will not always jump out at you or initially seem important. You may hear words, phrases, sentences, or intuit a complete knowing and understanding in a particular area of your health. Write down what you receive. If there are words that you see or hear and don't understand, look them up after the session.

It is likely that in addition to intuited thought-energy information, you will also experience a fair amount of mind chatter. This is normal. In the midst of the random thoughts, your intuitive receivers are still present and at work. Intuitive information will have energy—almost like a life of its own. You are not generating it from your personal thoughts. Intuitive energy information may feel imposed on you as if it wants to get your attention.

Intuited Feelings

The self-scan and the intuitive question exercise may trigger emotional release. You may recall memories, and suppressed sadness and grief may surface, or you may feel a knot of emotional energy letting go and not understand its origin or importance. Quite often just feeling the emotion is enough, as feeling it releases it.

Feel your emotions as they surface during the exercises, then document what you feel and any other energy information that you receive in relation to it.

If you are doing a scan for another, pay attention to the feelings that emerge. The emotional energy that you intuit from another may feel as if it is your own.

Intuited Body Sensations

Through the psychic skill of vibrational sensitivity and through your understanding of the chakras, the energy field, and the meridians, you will tune in to your body through a new perspective. Your body communicates to you through an array of intuitive sensations. You may feel an increase in energy, like a buzzing, moving through you. Certain areas of your body may feel dense or tight or in need of more medical attention. Your body may send you messages through images, feelings, and thoughts to eat better, exercise, or to lose weight. Messages may come in the form of inspiration or the motivation to get out and take a walk on a sunny day, or move your body through dance or another enjoyable activity.

Try to tune in to your bodily sensations as much as possible during intuitive work, even if what you experience makes no sense. Write down what you receive. Eventually you will better understand how your body communicates to you and be surprised by its wisdom and guidance.

When intuitively scanning another, remember to tune in to your physical sensations. This may likely be energy that you absorbed from another.

Intuited Images

Remember to trust your imagination when it comes to images that you receive during intuitive work. Your intuition and imagination work together to empower you to understand energy information.

Images may be symbolic, figurative, cartoonlike, or realistic-looking and three dimensional. At times you will "see" the organs and other systems of your physical body. These can be especially helpful. But, remember to also dialogue and ask questions of these images. No one kind of intuitive image is better than any other. It is only important that you understand and receive guidance from them.

Images can be seen with inner sight, felt, or sometimes we just know what they look like without a clear visual. You may also see energy through outer sight. Remember, ituitive sight is different than physical sight. It can encompass the specific intuitive input of all of the psychic skills.

Images are energy. Allow them to change, morph into new forms, and communicate with you. Try not to get stuck on how they appear. If you do not understand a particular image, ask to see it in a new way.

The Variety of Intuitive Guidance

Some of the messages you receive may not necessarily seem to be related to your health. You might receive a suggestion to avoid certain stressful situations, seek more solitude, and pursue a new occupation. You may suddenly feel the need to free yourself from a limiting relationship, speak your truth, and heal emotional wounds, or practice forgiveness and compassion. Although these issues may not seem to directly impact your health, they do. The root of good health is in your ability to stay in alignment with your true essence. When you are not in the flow of the power of your spirit, your health will eventually suffer in some way.

If you are intuitively scanning another, share all of the messages that you receive. Even if the intuited information does not seem necessarily health-related, or less than insightful and spectacular, it may be more meaningful than you know.

Let the energy information and images evolve over time.

Write down the energy information that you receive and it will continue to unfold and reveal new insights. Use the color charts to gain insight into any color energy that you see or sense. Refer back to the chakra information discussed in chapter 11 to gain more clarity and to better understand the emotional, mental, and spiritual challenges of each chakra and their physical association when you intuit energy information in these areas.

Expect to Continue to Receive Energy
Information When the Scan is Completed

Once the scan is completed you can investigate and gain more information about your health and the influences that are affecting it. Continue to ask yourself questions and intuitively listen within. The scan reveals unknown energy information. Once you have triggered this deeper knowing, it continues to surface long after the session is over.

Pay Attention to Your Dreams, Thoughts, and Feelings

Additional energy information may surface through your dreams or through intuitive feelings, thoughts, and an inner sense of knowing. Keep a journal of your scans and continue to document your dreams and other intuitive information that spontaneously surfaces.

Seek Help from Other Resources if Needed

If you encounter a physical issue or information that concerns you, consult with a physician or medical professional. Use the intuitive energy information that you have received to better equip you in getting additional help and support. If you become aware of suppressed memories, old traumas, or if difficult emotions or memories surface, consult a therapist or healer. Do not try to do everything yourself. There is no need to. Allow others to help and assist you in further healing.

If you are doing a scan for another, remember to refer them to medical professionals if it is indicated.

Other Types of Intuited Energy Information

Recognizing Past Life Influences

Past life influences can affect our health in a variety of ways. Some, who have had little to eat or starved to death in another life, have present-life food and eating disorder issues. If you were wounded or killed in battle in another life, you may have pain or a physical problem in the same area where you were wounded. Some of our fears, panic disorders, anxiety, and phobias trace back to difficulties and hardships that we have undergone in other lifetimes. We also at times limit ourselves and even suffer physical pain and disorders as a result of guilt over past life actions.

Understanding past lives can be surprisingly helpful in healing physical, emotional, mental, and spiritual disorders and diseases. While focusing on an area that may have lit up or felt hard or dense, if an image emerges that seems to be from another time or a different you, do not dismiss it. If an image emerges that you suspect may be a past life, simply ask the energy if this is so. You may hear, feel, or sense a response or visualize another confirming image. A past life will only emerge in a medical intuitive reading if it is important to present-time health and well-being. Listen to it. Close your eyes and remain open. Allow images to continue to emerge that will help you to understand that life. Continue to dialogue with the images.

Focus on what still may need healing and resolution from that life. Most importantly, ask the energy what you need to know in order to heal. Do not focus on the dates, the location, and other "interesting but not necessarily important for your health" information.

Once you have received all that you can about that life, ask for the energy of divine healing to flow through you. Release any feelings, guilt, stress, and fear that you may have had in that life. It is not important that you know everything that happened and fully understand it. It is more important to completely let go of the emotional energy connected with that life. Then forgive yourself and others. Open your heart and ask for the white light of source energy to fill the places in you where the past life emotional energy has been.

Past Life Influences in Others

If you are in the process of intuitively scanning another and you begin to see images that seem to be describing another time and place, allow them to unfold. Past life information generally will surface in a series of interconnected images. At times it may seem like you are viewing a movie. Pay attention to what emerges and use your other medical intuitive psychic skills to gain more information. Tell your client what you are receiving without filtering the content. If you are not sure it is a past life you are witnessing, tell this to your client. Whatever surfaces during a medical scan will in some way be related to health and well-being. Trust the process and be patient with understanding the significance.

How to Recognize and Release an Energy Attachment

During intuitive exercises if you come across any area that feels tight, dense, has a darkish or muted hue, and you cannot gain any information about it, you might have an energy attachment.

We do not like the idea that there are negative or unhealthy energy attachments that connect to our energy field and physical body. However, not being comfortable with this phenomena does not protect you from these potentially health-debilitating factors.

Energy attachments are rarely evil and powerful. You have full domain over your energy field and your physical body. Awareness is power. Once you know that there is an energy that is not yours robbing you of your energy and creating a block to you being able to fully accept and flow with vital life force source energy, you can easily remove it.

Energy attachments may be free-floating collective negative thought forms or emotions. They may be spirits who are lost in the astral plane who need a source of energy. Many positive and loving people attract these kinds of attachments because they are full of light and energy. Lost spirit attachments need a source of energy to fuel their existence in the lower vibrational levels. Once they ascend into the higher divine realms, they transform and are nourished by source energy.

Some attachments are aspects and split-off energy parts of people with whom you have been in relationship. These are family and friends and romantic partners who felt that they need you in order to survive. They may not want to let you go or they desire to control or possess you in some way. Through their unhealthy desires they unknowingly send a part of themselves to your energy field. Clinging onto you, an aspect of their energy attaches to you and drains your energy. Attachments can stifle your ability to feel free, confident, think for yourself, love another, and move forward in your life. Eventually an energy attachment will affect your physical health and sense of well-being.

Telltale Signs of Energy Attachments

If you persistently suffer from several of these symptoms and problems you may have an energy attachment.

- Fatigue

- Migraine headaches

- Physical conditions that resist healing

- Negative self-talk

- Exhaustion

- Weak immune system

- Frequent bouts of colds and the flu

- Psychosis

- Debilitating depression

- Nightmares

- Night sweats

- Obsessive behavior

- Unexplained physical pain

- Speaking words that make no sense

- Inability to move forward with your desires

- Crippling fear

- Phobias

- Free-floating stress and anxiety

MEDITATION: CLEARING

If you suspect that you have an energy attachment or simply want to be sure that you do not, this mediation will clear your energy field.

If you come across what appears to be an energy attachment while you are intuitively scanning another, you can guide him or her through this meditation.

INVOCATION OF LIGHT

Close your eyes. Breathe long, deep, relaxing breaths and release any stress and tension through the exhale.

Divine source of all of life; surround me
  with the white light of love and protection.

I invoke the highest love of all of creation to be
  above me, within me, by my side, within my heart,
  mind, body, and soul protecting and guiding me.

EXERCISE: ENERGY ATTACHMENT RELEASE

- Get into a comfortable position. You may want to lie down for this exercise. Close your eyes and take a long, deep breath, then exhale. Continue to breathe, sending the warm energy of the breath to any part of your body that is sore or tense or tight. Then breathe out all of the tension or stress. Continue with this cleansing breath. Each time you breathe, draw in warm and relaxing white light and exhale any tension from the body.

- Breathe in white light energy down through the top of your head. Exhale it through your heart. Continue breathing in white light and exhaling it through the heart. As you do this, imagine a white light bubble beginning to surround you. Continue to breathe as this bubble grows stronger and stronger. Imagine in this bubble of light that you are completely protected. Only what is in your highest good can enter.

- Send a prayer to the divine. This can be Archangel Michael, the Goddess, Mary, Jesus, the angelic realm, divine energy, or universal positive energy, whatever or whomever you feel a connection to. Ask for this being or energy to draw close and help you to release any negative energy or entity that is not in your highest good.

- Continue to breathe and imagine white light within your solar plexus. Breathe into this white light and imagine it expands as you exhale. Feel this white light as power. Breathe and expand this light of confidence and power. Imagine that it spreads out through your body and encompasses your energy field.

- As this light within you fully expands, imagine that any attachments or energy that is not yours shrivels and falls away. In its place white light enters and seals the area where it has been. Spend a few moments feeling the vibrancy of this luminous light surrounding you.

- When you feel that any energy attachments have been released, ask for the protection of white light to continue to repel anything from attaching to you that is not in your highest good.

- Imagine that you are surrounded by this white light of protection.

Taking the time to intuitively focus on your health is rewarding in many ways. Even though you may not always feel successful in your intuitive attempts to gain energy information, I assure you that you are doing more than you know to promote good health—mind, body, and spirit. Notice your successes and they will multiply. Every time you intuitively focus on your health, new layers of awareness and insights will surface.

In the next chapter you will learn the process for conducting a medical intuitive session.

14

HOW TO CONDUCT A
MEDICAL INTUITIVE SESSION

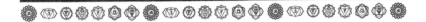

Intuiting the health of others and providing useful and practical guidance that empowers healing and increased well-being can be very rewarding. During the course of my many years as a professional psychic I have given readings in various areas of interest and concern. I have intuitively tuned in to energy information in areas such as relationship issues, finances, career opportunities, spirituality, and communication with angels and spirit guides. I am also a medium and communicate with those on the other side. Even though I have worked in various ways as a psychic, I was initially reluctant to use my intuitive ability in the area of health and wellness. Yet, during sessions, health and wellness energy information and guidance continued to emerge spontaneously. This natural occurrence, along with health-related questions from my clients, spurred on further study and a commitment to focus on medical intuition.

To my surprise it has been through medical intuitive work that I have discovered and learned the most about who we are and the nature of reality. Medical intuition has opened my heart, my mind, and my soul. It has helped me to stay healthy and enjoy close feelings of connection to those in the physical and spiritual worlds. When you help others through your natural intuitive ability you not only better understand our interconnectedness with one another and with the all that is, you live it as a day-to-day reality.

Ethical Considerations

There is no governing board of ethics or agreed upon ethical standards in the field of medical intuition. Yet, it is vital to have a personal code of ethics that guides your work with others. Acting in integrity, being authentic, maintaining good boundaries, and being respectful of self and others plays a major role in your success as a medical intuitive and in the healing work itself.

Medical intuition demands higher ethical standards than other forms of intuitive work. Allowing another to tune in to your thoughts, feelings, physical body, and spiritual energy is an act of trust. Your client should be treated with kindness, compassion, and intuitive honesty.

A Sacred Contract

There is an unspoken sacred contract between yourself and your client. You are being invited into the deep recess of another's body, mind, and spirit. Act as a messenger of love, wisdom, and insight. Always intend to do your best and intuit energy information for the highest good.

Treat Others with Respect

There are a few temptations that will likely arise as you become more confident with your intuitive skills. It can be a bit of a thrill to intuitively tune in to another and receive important energy information. Feelings of power and accomplishment often accompany correct intuitive insights. Remember that the care of your client is your priority. It may be tempting to focus on your intuitive successes instead of the vulnerable person who sits before you. People may come to you feeling ignored or confused by the health care system. They are likely nervous and feel that their innermost fears and thoughts will be exposed. Tread lightly and always with the highest motivation and intent. Be kind, loving, and compassionate.

Get Permission

It might also be tempting to intuitively tune in to others without their permission. Even though it is possible to do this, train yourself to activate your intuition only when asked. Although you might have energy information that you feel will help another, do not confront others with what you may have randomly intuitively received. Instead, send an intuitive message to the person and their angels. If what you have naturally received is important for him or her to know, ask that the person approach you and ask for your input. If this does not happen, imagine the person surrounded by white, healing light energy and send them a prayer for their highest good and healing.

It is also important that you never share or discuss another's medical or personal information with anyone without their permission. You may have had an enlightening and gratifying session where you intuitively pinpointed the cause of an illness or disease in another. You may want to tell others and even post it on your website. Remember the insights you receive are to help your client. Always get your client's permission before you share information about a session with others.

Maintain Good Boundaries

Maintain good boundaries with your clients and with your friends and family members. Resist the temptation to be available for their every concern and issue. Although you may want to be lovingly supportive, helpful, and present to others in every way possible, you will slowly take their power away if you do this. Do not put yourself in the position of becoming another's source of constant intuitive medical insight and information. As a medical intuitive it is important to support others' intuitive self-awareness and not replace it with your own. Support and encourage your clients to trust their own intuition. Be a source of empowerment for others by reinforcing their ability to listen within and make good health choices.

Your friends and family members will likely want you to tune in to their health concerns. Even if they have initially voiced their doubt and concerns, they may seek your advice and insight. If you do choose to intuitively work with a loved one, try to remain as objective as possible. It is also important not to become entangled in relationship and personality drama and issues. I prefer to refer those who are close to me to other intuitive and health care professionals.

Criticism and Rejection

Clients who are ill, in pain, or confused about their health can be nervous, sensitive, fearful, and reactive. At times they may dispute or be critical of the energy information that you intuit. If this happens to you, listen to your client's concerns. Do not allow your ego to take over and become defensive. At the same time it is important to treat yourself with respect and not become a dumping ground for another's stress and fear. If the client becomes negative and overly critical, let him or her know that you are open to feedback and input that is helpful and constructive. Do not argue with a client who does not agree with your intuitive findings. Be respectful of their right to view their health in the way that they choose to. Maintain poise and support the client in their feelings without taking responsibility for another's negativity, feelings of frustration, or stress.

There are times when it is difficult to accurately intuitively tune in to another's health. This happens for many reasons. Sometimes the client is so fearful that they put a defensive energy wall around themselves that is difficult to intuitively penetrate. It might also be possible that you are over tired, or it may be in your client's highest good to gain insight about their health through another avenue.

We all make mistakes and misread or misinterpret the energy information. This is natural and it will happen. Consider those times that you are incorrect in your intuitive evaluation to be a useful learning experience. Do not become overly self-critical, call yourself a failure, and take it too personally. Try to understand what you misread or misinterpreted. If you approach it in this way, you will likely not make this error again.

Remember that a medical intuitive session is not a doctor examination. Listen to the heart and soul of your client. Respond with a loving and kind attitude. In this way, healing is always present.

Be an Example of Health and Wellness

Being a medical intuitive is more than an interesting job. It is a daily devotion to living in integrity and mind, body, and spirit health and self-awareness. Eat healthy foods, get plenty of rest, and listen and act on your own intuitive health messages. Meditate and challenge limiting and negative thoughts, heal your emotional wounds, forgive others, and do all that you can do to maintain your serenity and inner peace. Self-awareness is an important part of intuitive work as it clears the channels for the entrance of divine guidance, love, and wisdom. Be willing to put the time and effort into being, healing, and growing, and evolving mind, body, and spirit.

Living a healthy life—mind, body, and spirit—will not only set a good example for your clients, it will also prevent you from projecting your own unresolved issues and needs into medical intuitive sessions.

Healing as a Part of the Session

When you are able to identify and help another through medical intuition, you will likely be asked and at times expected to also heal the problems and issues that you uncover. It can be a temptation to attempt to be all and do all. Know your limitations and get to know other healers and practitioners that you can confidently recommend to others.

If you are interested in offering other healing modalities such as Reiki, healing touch, emotional release, hypnotherapy, herbal medicine, etc., inform your client that you also work in these modalities and offer to set up a separate appointment in an area that he or she may want to explore. Do not include specific healing modalities in a medical intuition session unless you have informed the client ahead of time that you are going to include it and they are comfortable with this.

Legal Considerations

It is illegal to practice medicine without a medical license. In the area of holistic health and alternative healing practices, laws and regulations vary from location to location. Medical intuition is an ever-evolving practice with new discoveries and positive results increasing on a daily basis. Keep up with the current laws in your area. As science catches up in being able to prove the validity and usefulness of medical intuition, regulations are bound to change.

It is advisable not to promise or guarantee any specific healing and health-related outcome and result. Be careful not to make any medical claims or contracts (even verbal) of accuracy in diagnoses. Medical intuition is the ability to access and communicate health-related energy information. Know your limits. There are many factors and influences that go into creating an accurate and successful session. As much as you may want to help another, healing occurs when a client is ready and willing to heal and act in their highest good.

Release Form

Some medical intuitives ask their clients to sign a release form. If you decide to do this, keep it simple. A release form should clearly state that your role is as an intuitive energy consultant and not a medical professional. This can be helpful in a few different ways. This eliminates false expectations and legally protects you. You may want to consult with an attorney in your area to discuss a binding agreement. A medical intuitive release form can be simply stated and may look something like this.

I _____(client's name) understand that _____(your name) is an intuitive energy specialist and consultant and not a medical doctor, a medically trained practitioner, licensed, certified, or registered nurse, or medical professional. (If you are a medical doctor, nurse, or medical professional, state that you are working with the client as an intuitive medical energy specialist.)

_____(your name) has not offered me any medical or health-related expectations, false promises, and assurances of certain outcomes. I _____(client's name) further understand that a medical intuitive reading is not a substitute for a consultation with a medical doctor.

X_____(client signature)

Setting Fees

Most people who become medical intuitives are motivated by a desire to help and be of service to others. Yet, charging a fee for your services will at some point be necessary. If you are unsure that you want to give medical intuitive readings to others, or if you are beginning to develop medical intuition and not feeling completely confident with your skills, it is fine to do readings at no cost. Be sure to explain to others that you are a beginner or that you desire to practice giving readings.

If you are ready to practice medical intuition in a more public way, it will be necessary to set a fee or make the decision to work on a sliding scale or a donation basis. Whatever avenue you choose is a personal decision. Consider your experience, the amount of time that you will devote to a session, the fee that other alternative health care practitioners charge in your area, and most importantly what you feel comfortable with.

Charging a fee, working on a sliding scale, or accepting donations will ensure more successful sessions. We tend to value and are more receptive when we contribute in some way. Money is a form of energy. Your client will be more invested in the session when there is a fee. Paying for sessions creates an energetic give-and-take balance between yourself and your client.

In-Person and Long-Distance Sessions

Some medical intuitives prefer to work with their clients in person and do not do phone work, while others prefer phone sessions. Some clients prefer in-person sessions but will do fine with phone work if you express confidence with this option. The quality of a medical intuitive session is determined more by the client's openness and confidence with the intuitive process rather than their physical presence. One of the benefits of medical intuition is that you do not have to be physically present to give an accurate health analysis. At times phone readings can be more accurate as the appearance of the physical body can be misleading. Energy is not limited to time and space. As you become more comfortable with communicating with energy, you will find that it is always responsive and reliable no matter where you are.

Preparing the Client

Decide how much you want to know about your client's health before a session and ask them to share only this with you. I don't ask for any health information before I begin. But this is a personal decision and it's important to find what works for you.

Ask your client not to drink alcohol for twenty-four hours previous to the session and not to eat for at least an hour before the session. While viewing the digestive system can be fascinating, spending time viewing what someone had for lunch is probably not the best use of time and energy.

For phone sessions ask your client to sit in a quiet room where they can be undisturbed, with uncrossed legs and feet on the floor during the session. This aids in accurately reading the flow of energy through the body. It's surprising how many people have asked me to do health readings while they are driving or sitting outside of their workplace eating lunch. A calm atmosphere will help you to stay focused during the length of time that a medical reading requires. Keep yourself hydrated by drinking water during the session.

Before you begin the session tell your client what to expect. Tell him or her how you will begin and then proceed through the medical scan. Communicate what you receive as you receive it. Once you have completed the process and have shared your intuitive impressions, ask the client if they have any questions.

Meditation: Clearing

During a medical intuitive session it is important not to absorb any of your client's health issues or imbalanced energy into your body. This is one reason I suggest you dialogue with energy and use images to perceive and intuit a client's health. In addition, I suggest you use the following quick clearing and protection meditation before you begin a session.

Close your eyes and imagine breathing white light energy down through the top of the head. Continue to breathe white light energy breaths. Slowly move the white light breath through your entire body. Exhale any negativity, stress, and tension, and ask that it be lifted and transformed with the light of divine energy. Continue to breathe in white light and release any stress, negativity, or tension. Once you have sent white light through the entire body imagine this light completely encompassing you. This light allows only what is in your highest good to enter and it repels any negative or harmful energy. Ask for your spirit helpers to be present to assist and further protect you from unwanted energy influences.

Prayer

After you have completed the silent meditation, you may want to say a prayer or invoke divine presence. You might want to use something like this:

Mother, Father God (divine presence, universal life source energy, etc., whatever you are comfortable with) as we draw close we ask for the white light of your love and protection. We also ask for any of (client's name) healing and helping angels, and loved ones on the other side that can provide useful health information, wisdom, and healing energy to draw close. We ask for insight and guidance that will further (client's name) emotional, mental, spiritual, and physical health and well-being.

Dialogue with the Energy

During a medical intuitive session it is important to focus on communicating with the client's energy. You will likely initially begin to receive intuitive information through your primary intuitive type—mental, emotional, physical, or spiritual. However your intuition surfaces, ask to see the energy in an image on a blank screen. Using this method allows you to dialogue with the client's energy and higher vibration sources of guidance without absorbing the client's energy. It will also enable you to receive intuitive information in a more comprehensive way. In time, this process will become natural and be a consistently reliable way to gain trustworthy energy information. Remember, your intuition and imagination work together. If it feels like you are making up an image, go with this. If it is an authentic representation of the energy it will continue to unfold and reveal energy information.

Focus on and ask for more information if an image of an area lights up, has a buzzing feel or sound, or if you feel a hardened or inert energy flow. If an image does not light up and the energy flows smoothly, move on to the next area. If an image lights up or if you feel a hardness or inertia in the energy flow, this is an indication that there is a dysfunction or problem. In this case ask to see another image of the problem area. Once you perceive an image of the problem area, ask the following questions one at a time, and then ask for an image that will provide you with the information. If you do not understand the image, ask for another image, thought, or emotional insight for clarification.

Questions to ask the energy images:

- *How is this energy manifesting in the body?*

- *If this energy had a voice what would it be saying?*

- *What is the emotional energy connected to this image?*

- *What is the spiritual message connected to this issue or area?*

Not all of these questions will be answered. The ones that are important for the area of the body that you are scanning will have more energy. This may feel like a tingle, or you may see a sparkle of light. In time you will be better able to discern the presence of important energy information.

Receiving Intuitive Information

Use your psychic skills of clairvoyance, clairsentience, claircognizance, clairaudience, and vibrational sensitivity to tune in to the energy information that you are given. Some of these questions will elicit more information than others. If you ask one of these questions and the image that emerges lacks energy and quickly fades, move on to the next question.

Describe to your client the energy images that you receive. You will likely receive symbolic, figurative, and realistic images of organs and bodily systems. I have found that describing the physical realistic images of the body that I intuit to be especially helpful to the client in understanding what is happening in their body. Remember to communicate and ask questions of the more realistic images as well.

Along with an image you may receive energy information as spontaneous knowing, awareness of your client's emotional wounds, pain, beliefs, and attitudes that are affecting their health or soul plan. You may also hear words and phrases. If you hear a word that you do not understand write it down and later look it up in a medical dictionary. After you understand the meaning of the word, contact your client and share it with him or her. Sometimes I receive more intuitive information after I am finished with a session. If this happens to you, contact your client and share what you received.

One of the most common questions that I am asked by intuitive development students is how to discern intuitive energy information from ego thoughts and feelings. Energy information will be calm, persistent, and give you a consistent message. During readings I know that I have not thoroughly described or received intuitive information if it does not move out of my consciousness. Unlike the ego voice that chatters away and can be emotionally charged and self-centered, intuitive information is quiet but relentless.

During the session describe to your client what you are receiving. Do not filter or try to figure out or over-analyze. Do not attempt to prematurely diagnose an issue or problem. When I intuit an illness such as cancer or another life-threatening illness, I describe as best as I can what I perceive in the area. I tell the client that it's important that they see a doctor as soon as possible. Sometimes a client will ask me if they have cancer. If they do, I tell them that I feel a tumor or other telltale signs of this. But, again I insist that they get this checked out by a medical doctor. If you hear the word *cancer* or another disease or illness, continue to dialogue with the energy and ask for confirming energy evidence.

As a medical intuitive your responsibility is to describe as accurately as possible the energy information that you receive. People will often want a quick diagnosis. Resist the temptation to rush the intuitive process. Explain as accurately as you can what you intuit without trying to label a specific illness or disease. Often what you describe will be more important to your client than what he or she initially believes. If you are unclear of the meaning of what you are receiving tell this to your client and still describe what you are receiving as best as you can.

Refer back to the last chapter for more intuitive interpretation guidelines.

Speak with Compassion

Medical intuitive sessions are like surgery on the soul. Your client is vulnerable and in need of love, safety, and compassion. They may be in pain, frightened, and confused as to the state of their health. Words are powerful, and it is important to share what you receive in a supportive, nonaccusatory way. Otherwise, they will withdraw their energy and try to block your intuitive perception. Medical intuitive sessions provide an opportunity for immense healing. You want your client to feel understood and acknowledged. Your aim should be always to support your client and help them to feel safe and supported. Allow your client to accept or reinterpret your intuitive impressions. Resist the temptation to be "right."

Communicate what you receive with compassion and "I" statements.

Instead of saying: "You are angry "or "Your negative attitude is making you sick." Say something like: "I feel anger or sadness in your stomach." Or, "My intuitive impression is that negative energy is impacting your health."

If you see images of your client in a difficult experience, for instance, an image of him or her being abused as a child or an image that you suspect is a past life where they suffered or caused others pain, be careful how you describe what you receive.

Instead of saying, "You were abused as a child by your father," or "You are in pain because you caused others pain in another life," say something like: "I see an image of a child. It appears to be you. I feel abuse and pain in this image." Or, "My intuitive impression is that there is unfinished business from a past life that is affecting your health."

Then describe the image that you receive in "I" statements, such as, "This is what I see … this is what I feel … this is the thought that came to me."

Allow your client to accept, reject, or reinterpret your intuitive insight. Sometimes it takes a little while to take in all the information that they are receiving. A client may feel a bit overwhelmed. Give him or her space and do not expect affirmation and confirmation on all that you receive.

After the Session

Develop a routine after and in between sessions and stick to it. It is important to take the time to come into balance and restore your energy after working with another. Drink water, get up, stretch your legs, and breathe deeply or take a walk. Do whatever helps you to let go of any energy you have intuited and absorbed, and to feel centered.

EXERCISE: INTUITIVE SCAN FOR ANOTHER

Scanning others is similar to the process of scanning yourself. Here is the method that I recommend. Begin this method after you say a protection prayer and invite your spirit helpers into the reading.

- Focus your awareness in the client's seventh chakra. This is slightly above the client's head. Breathe a long deep breath and relax. Imagine an energy spiral above your client's head. Ask to view this energy spiral on a blank screen. Notice its colors and texture; feel the vibrational flow of energy move through it.

- Once you have viewed an image of the energy spiral above your client's head, ask for the spiral to spread out to the width of their energy field. Imagine this spiral of energy as four sections, which extend upwards from the front, side, back, and other side of your client's head.

  1. Begin to scan this section by section in a clockwise motion. Ask for an image of each section one at a time. If the area lights up, has a slight buzz, or if you feel an inertia or hardness in the energy flow, ask to see an image of the problem area.

  2. Questions to ask the image:
     - *How is this energy manifesting in the body?*
     - *If this energy had a voice what would it be saying?*
     - *What is the emotional energy connected to this image?*
     - *What is the mental thought energy or beliefs and attitudes associated with this area?*
     - *What is the spiritual message connected to this issue or area?*

  3. Not all of the questions will be answered. The ones that are important for the area of the body that you are scanning will have more energy. This may feel like a tingle or you may see a sparkle of light. Communicate to your

client what you are receiving. You have sufficiently and thoroughly received all of the information when the area that you are viewing no longer lights up or tingles or has a buzzing feel. It will emit a calm, toned-down energy that no longer is trying to get your attention and is beginning to fade. When this happens move onto the next section.

- Once you have completed all four sections of the expanded seventh chakra energy spiral, you will now scan the energy field. Starting at the seventh chakra above the head, imagine the energy field completely surrounding the client's body. Segment the energy field into four sections: front, right side, back, and then left side. Scan one section at a time in a vertical manner, asking for an image of each section. If a section lights up, tingles, or if you feel inertia or hardened energy, ask to see an image of the problem area and then proceed with steps one through three.

- When you have completed all four sections of the energy field, move your awareness to the sixth chakra. Become aware of a spiral of energy in the center of the client's head. Ask the energy to encompass the entire head and expand a few inches outside of the head. Segment the energy field into four sections: the brain, sinus and face, eyes and nose, and then ears and teeth.

- Scan one section at a time, asking for an image of each section. If a section lights up, tingles, or if you feel inertia or hardened energy, ask to see an image of the problem area and then proceed with steps one through three. Describe as best you can what you receive to your client. When a section no longer lights up move onto the next section.

- When you have completed scanning the sixth chakra move your awareness to the client's fifth chakra, the throat area.

Ask the energy to expand to encompass the throat and shoulder and arms. Segment this area into the neck, the throat, the shoulders, and the arms and hands. If a section lights up, tingles, or if you feel inertia or hardened energy, ask to see an image of the problem area and then continue with steps one through three.

- Once you have scanned this area move your awareness to the fourth chakra, the chest area. Feel the energy spiral of the fourth chakra. Ask for this energy to expand and include the heart and lung area. Expand this energy a few inches outside of the body. Divide the chest area into the heart, bronchial tubes, lungs, and breasts. Ask for an image to appear on the blank screen that represents the energy of each area one at a time. If an image lights up, tingles, or feels hardened and inert, ask for an image that represents the problem. Continue with steps one through three.

- When you have completed scanning the client's chest area, move your awareness to the solar plexus. Imagine an energy spiral within the abdomen. Expand this spiral to encompass the entire area and extending about two inches outside of the body. Separate this area into the stomach, gallbladder, liver, spleen, and then the pancreas.

- Scan each section one at a time. Again, as in previous sections, ask for an image of each section, if it lights up or feels hardened or inert, ask for an image of the problem and continue with steps one through three.

- Once you have completed the solar plexus scan move your awareness to a few inches below the navel. Imagine a spiral of energy within the client's body and ask this energy spiral to expand to encompass the entire area including a few inches outside of the body. Separate this area into the colon, which lies across the stomach, the right and left ovaries and uterus for women, the bladder low center, and for men, the prostate.

- Scan each section one at a time. Again, as in previous sections, ask for an image of each section. If it lights up, tingles, or feels hardened or inert, ask for an image of the problem and continue with steps one through three.

- When you have completed scanning this section, move your awareness to the lower part of the client's body. Imagine a spiral of energy within the body and ask for this spiral to expand to encompass the entire lower part of the body. Separate this area into the spine, the right and left kidney, the lower colon, and the legs and the feet. Scan each section one at a time. Ask for an image of each section, if it lights up, tingles, or feels hardened or inert, ask for an image of the problem and continue with steps one through three.

- When you have completed scanning this section, move your awareness to a spot a few inches below the pubic bone. Intend to scan the endocrine system. Ask for an image of each gland. Begin with the ovaries if you are working with a woman and the testes if you working with a man. When you have scanned the ovaries or testes, ask for an image of the adrenals, then the thymus, thyroid, pituitary, and then the pineal. Ask for an image to appear on the blank screen that represents the energy of each area one at a time. If an image lights up, tingles, or feels hardened and inert, ask for an image that represents the problem. Continue with steps one through three.

- When you have completed each gland, ask for an image that includes the energy of the glands flowing in unison. Scan this image. If this image does not light up or draw your attention in any way, you have completed this area. If it does light up, ask for an image of the problem or issue, then ask questions to further understand the problem.

- Move your attention back down to the soles of the client's feet. Imagine a spiral of energy and ask this energy to expand through the entire body and extend several inches outside of the body. Ask to view the lymphatic, the circulatory, the nervous, and the skeletal systems one at a time. Ask for an image of each section. If an area lights up, tingles, or buzzes, or feels hardened or inert, ask for additional information and proceed with steps one through three. Scan each section in this way.

- Ask your client if they have any questions. If they ask for more information about a specific area or share an issue that you have not detected, draw your awareness to the area of their concern and ask for an image. Continue with steps one through three. Share what you receive. Sometimes clients will want definitive answers and become frustrated if they are not hearing what they want to hear. Remain calm and focused on the energy. Be compassionate without being tempted to exceed your abilities. Describe what you receive and be sure to recommend that the client follow up with medical professionals.

- When you have completed this scan, imagine a spiral of energy at the top of your client's head. Ask divine healing energy to enter this energy spiral. Ask that this energy spiral of white light healing energy move through your client's entire body and energy field. Breathe, take your time, and allow this energy to move through your client, healing and cleansing and revitalizing your client—mind, body, and spirit. When you have completed this energy healing, imagine a white light orb of energy completely surrounding your client.

- Thank your spirit helpers, angels, and the divine for their presence, help, and healing. Send them love and gratitude.

If you have detected any illness, dysfunction, or disease, ask the client to follow up with conventional and alternative medical professionals' help. Encourage the client to address and heal any emotional wounds that you have uncovered. If you have detected any energy attachments or past lives that you feel need further examination and healing, suggest that your client follow up with a reputable practitioner that can address these issues. It can be helpful to network with medical doctors, energy healers, massage therapists, hypnotherapists, chiropractors, naturopaths, acupuncturists, and other types of practitioners and healers that you can recommend to your clients if they need a referral.

A Sample Scan

Every medical intuitive reading is different. Some empathize physical issues, others reveal more emotional, mental, and spiritual issues. I offer you this example of a session to give you an idea of a medical intuitive reading. Your sessions will most likely differ in many ways from this.

Stacy was referred to me by an acupuncturist for a medical intuitive reading. She lives in California and I am in North Carolina so our phone session was a bit early in the morning for her. Most people want to have readings in the evening and on the weekend to accommodate their schedule. Yet, early morning is the best time for a reading. The mind is clear, we are rested, and the energetic vibrations are active and easily accessible.

I begin phone sessions in the same way as an in-person session. I do a short clearing of my energy and then say a prayer, inviting the divine presence and my spirit helpers and angels to be present.

As I began to tune in to Stacy's aura at the top of her head I felt an angel guiding and communicating with me. The energy above her head immediately lit up. After asking to see an image of this area, I saw a division in the flow of energy coming from her aura into her seventh chakra. Soon after this image another one spontaneously emerged without asking for it. At some point after using this medical intuitive process the energy will respond automatically without your conscious request.

In the image that spontaneously emerged there is an older man crouched over a desk hard at work. I had the claircognizance knowing that this was Stacy in another life. Sending a silent message to the energy, I asked for more information. I quickly received a flood of thoughts that I shared with Stacy.

I told her, "As soon as I began to tune in to your energy, I felt a division in the flow of vital life force energy coming into your body. Your male and female energy is unbalanced. I see a past life image of you as a man. I get the intuitive impression that you were very devoted to your work. It feels to me that you have had many lives as a male focused in the area of science and medicine. I hear the message that in this life you are meant to explore your more feminine side. Intuition, creativity, and putting energy into relationships is important. The right side of your body is your male energy. It is strong. But the left side, which is your female energy, is weaker. This is causing some physical issues that I will further investigate as we continue. "

Continuing with the scan I asked for images of the rest of her energy field. When none lit up or drew my attention I began to scan the head area. Again I was not alerted and I moved down to the neck and shoulder area. When I asked for an image of the back of her neck, it lit up. In the next image I saw a close-up of the upper cervical neck area. It was red and I could feel pain and swelling. I asked for more information and I heard that there had been a recent and past accident that affected this area.

I shared with Stacy, "As I come into the lower neck area I feel pain. It feels to me that you had a few accidents that have affected this area, one in the past and another not too long ago. I feel swelling and pain."

"Yes, that's correct," Stacy confirmed. "I ran my bike into a wall when I was a kid. It knocked the wind out of me and injured my neck. Then several months ago, I was in a car accident. The pain will not go away. I am not healing as fast as I expected to."

I continued with the scan. The next area image also lit up. This was in the thyroid area. After asking for another image, I saw that the thyroid was thick and a little larger on the left side. The energy flow felt stifled. I shared this with Stacy and told her that I would need to scan the endocrine system to fully understand what was going on in the thyroid.

I decided to continue scanning her body in order before focusing on the endocrine system. I moved my intuitive awareness into her chest area. When I scanned the left side of her chest I was alerted. I asked for an image and saw heavy, swollen tissue. When I asked for more information, I saw an enlarged image of the left side of her body. The energy flow was stagnant and this was causing edema. Asking questions to discern the influences of this condition, I felt a sense of loss and sadness.

I shared with Stacy. "There is some edema on the left side of your body. I am feeling relationship loss and stress. I see you trying to communicate with a woman. I feel as if you are not being heard and understood. This seems to be strengthening one of the underlying challenges of this life, developing your feminine energy and relationship communication."

"I have been having some trouble with my two sisters and my mother," Stacy told me. "I'm not sure what is going on. My younger sister confronted me about a past issue a few months ago and is no longer talking to me. My other sister is sympathetic to her. My mother says she doesn't want to get involved, but I think that she is stirring up trouble behind my back. It's been very painful for close to a year now."

I continued to scan her body. When I got to the left hip and knee area I was alerted by an image that lit up. As I communicated with the dull blue and red energy images of this area, I realized that the soreness I felt here was connected to an accident. Most likely this was the recent car accident. I shared this with Stacy and she confirmed my findings. The accident bruised her left hip area and she had been going to physical therapy for it.

I scanned the endocrine system and I was alerted by a heavy feeling and a muddy brown color. I also did a meridian check of this area to better understand the energy flow. The endocrine system controls the flow of life-giving source energy through the body and can be extremely informative in understanding subtle but significant health issues. I was alerted and continued to ask for images and to dialogue with the energy.

I told Stacy, "I feel that the energy movement through the adrenals and ovaries and then up to the thyroid and pineal and pituitary gland is flowing in irregular waves. This is causing an array of issues. Your sleep feels interrupted. Some nights you may sleep deep and some you may have insomnia. Your metabolism is also up and down and your hormones are fluctuating. When I ask for the origin of this issue I am led back to where I began. There is an imbalance between the feminine and masculine flow of energy throughout your body. The endocrine system moves energy into every organ and bodily system. It is the body's energy brain. The thyroid helps to transform higher vibration source energy into nutrition for the organs and other bodily systems. I feel as if your thyroid is struggling to regulate the up and down inflow of energy. The result is feelings of exhaustion and at other times you probably feel like you are crawling out of your skin with too much energy."

Stacy sat in deep thought and then told me, "The reason I made this appointment was to see what you would say about my thyroid and neck. Since the accident my neck seems to hurt all the time, despite weekly physical therapy, acupuncture, and massages. Nothing seems to help the pain. But that's not all. I guess I can tell you this and you won't think that I'm crazy. I woke up early one morning and was lying in bed in a half-awake state when I heard this voice. It felt like it was coming from me, but it was not really me. The voice told me to have my thyroid checked. I have been gaining weight recently so I went to see my doctor. He told me that it is enlarged and he gave me an array of tests, but they all came out normal. Is there a connection between my neck and my thyroid? If my thyroid is fine, why did I hear this voice?"

"We talked about the injuries in your neck and your need for continued massage and acupuncture. As we just discussed your endocrine system is struggling as a result of an imbalance in your masculine and feminine energy flow. The thyroid in particular is having a difficult time converting this energy into useable physical nutrition. To answer your question, there is an energetic connection between the two." I told her, "Your neck and the thyroid gland are both located in the fifth chakra. This chakra represents the voice of our authentic self. When I tune in to your fifth chakra energy I see an image of you struggling to be heard and understood by your family. I feel that one of your life lessons is to fully embrace and express your true self. I know that you have felt rejected by your sisters. But you cannot control how they respond and react to you. This is out of your control. Don't measure yourself by how your family accepts you. I know that this is not always easy to do. Know that your responsibility is to you. I get the message that it would be good for you to seek out friends, especially women that give you positive support and are able to see and know who you are. Your guides are telling me that you were alerted about your thyroid before it became a medical issue. You can heal this issue while it is still an energy imbalance and avoid any future issues."

I continued with the scan and was not alerted to any other issues. I finished by visualizing white light source energy moving through her body from the top of her head to the soles of her feet. As I did this I felt her energy shift from an irregular disjointed flow to a more vibrant flowing current. I asked my healing angels to widen the flow of feminine energy into her seventh chakra. I finished by visualizing healing green and white energy in her throat area.

When I am finished with the medical intuitive session, I like to take a few moments before my next client to clear my energy. I drink water and, if I have time, I take a short walk.

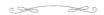

Giving medical intuitive readings to others is an honor and a privilege. Be mindful of others' vulnerabilities. Even slight suggestions and certain phrasing of intuited feedback is likely to have an effect. View your work as a medical intuitive as a gift from a greater source of love and wisdom. Be the conduit from which another will gain not only valuable energy health-related information, but feel compassion, caring, and kindness as well.

The next chapter explores a few other ways that intuition emerges in our lives and how to connect with higher helpful energies.

Section 5

MORE TOOLS FOR THE MEDICAL INTUITIVE MEDICINE BAG

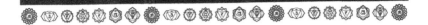

WORKING WITH SPIRIT HELPERS

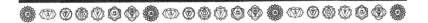

Becoming a medical intuitive is a step into evolutionary spiritual awareness. Your efforts to evolve and move in to your authentic power as a medical intuitive do not happen in a vacuum. It is a journey that you will never travel alone. As you activate your innate intuitive ability to heal self and others, benevolent universal power becomes an active force in your life. The intuitive awareness that you are developing is not just for you. As you progress along this path, you spontaneously attract opportunities to become a positive force for others and for the earth. There is a magical magnetism that is always in operation. Let go of your ego fears and limited thinking, listen within to your intuition, take responsibility, and act in integrity. As you participate in life in this way, a beam of light within you sends out a signal to those you can help.

Help from the Spirit Realm

One of the most exciting aspects of becoming a medical intuitive is the inner intuitive assurance that you are part of a powerful celestial network of wisdom, healing, and love. When you claim the power of your spirit, you activate your multidimensional connection to vast resources of love, wisdom, and healing. Even when you feel as if you are alone and question your abilities, your efforts are being recognized and supported in the higher realms of spirit.

The paradigm of medical intuition employs universal life force wisdom, love, and healing energy. You work in unison with the healing energies of the earth and the heavens. Not only do you spontaneously attract individuals in the physical world that you can help and who can help you, you also attract spiritual helpers.

When I began to deepen and refine my medical intuitive abilities, I had a surprising encounter with a spirit guide who let me know of his intention to assist me in my work. One of my meditative practices is going to the local pool and swimming laps. I have done this for years. The rhythmic back and forth motion of the water is a continuous source of inspiration and new ideas. One morning while swimming I did a turn at one end of the pool and abruptly stopped and stood up. I felt as if I had hit an invisible wall. As I stood there for a moment feeling curiously stunned, I heard an authoritative voice say: "I am Dr. Roshi. You are fortunate. I have decided to work with you and help you."

My connection with spirit guides and angels goes back to my youth. I have always relied on their presence and help in my intuitive work. But never before have I experienced such a formal introduction to a spirit guide. I thanked him and listened for more guidance. None came. As quickly as I felt his presence stop me, he was gone. However, I knew he would be back.

Soon after this, I was giving a health reading to a client and sure enough, I again felt Dr. Roshi's abrupt and strong presence. From the advice and guidance he gave to me, I knew that he must have been listening in during the session.

Over the years Dr. Roshi's advice and perspective has been invaluable. Not a warm and fuzzy guide, he is all business and his input is clear and to the point. I imagine he may be busy in other endeavors as he usually seems a bit rushed and even at times impatient with me. Yet, I have learned quite a bit from Dr. Roshi. For instance, he taught me to observe the body horizontally as well as vertically. A rotating position, he informed me, is a better way to discern the energy that surrounds the body. His expertise is in teaching and encouraging me to understand the connection between our health and the energy of the earth and heavens. This includes the body's organic balance with the natural elements. His view is always interesting and usually surprising. Yet, his insight and wisdom always proves to be reliable.

Balancing the Elements

In a recent session, Dr. Roshi offered an interesting explanation for a client's physical health issues. Annie is a spiritual seeker in her late fifties. A single woman, she travels quite a bit and enjoys various spiritual practices. When I did a health scan for her, I became aware of weakness in her lower body, especially her knees. Her tendency to retain fluids was beginning to cause joint pain and other problems. As I explained what I was receiving, she asked me for Dr. Roshi's advice. In other sessions I shared his insight with her, which she seemed to benefit from. I sent an inner request to him and he was suddenly present.

In his crisp, no-nonsense kind of way, he told me, "Annie is like a weeping willow. She is grounding her energy deep into the earth. But she is absorbing too much of the water element. Her legs and hips are soggy, and the dampness, it is seeping into her joints and beginning to cause problems. She goes outside of herself, into the world for love. Trying to fill her heart and body with love from an incorrect source, the love she seeks can only be found within. Her heart is absorbing too much external emotional energy and this is causing an imbalance with the water element. Annie needs to ground her energy with the sun. The sun rays will add fire to mind, body, and spirit—help her to become stronger and let go of the fluid that she is drowning in. For her heart, she must have courage and determination to find the love she seeks within self."

Intent, Action, Integrity

To develop your medical intuitive abilities to their highest potential and to attract celestial help, it is necessary to have a sense of clear intent and purpose. Intent is more than an interesting concept. Your intent constructs and defines your energy pattern. It sends out a call to the universe declaring what you desire to receive and manifest. When you develop medical intuition you are essentially building an energetic pathway of interconnectedness between the mind, body, emotions, spirit, and the vast network of cosmic wisdom and love. This energy path empowers you to tune in to your own and others' health and well-being. Your intuition begins to operate like an unseen-energy MRI or X-Ray machine with celestial benefits.

If you want to develop medical intuition to impress your friends, control others, or make a lot of money, then your efforts will not be supported by the highest energetic source. When your intent is to be of service, embody the truth of your being, and share and receive love and positivity, then your efforts are supported by powerful celestial forces. You cannot fool the heavens.

Along with intent comes action. Become clear as to what your reasons are for developing your intuition and act on this intent. In both significant, and what appear to be insignificant ways, you will be given the opportunity to put this awareness into action. This does not only apply to intuitive work. Be of service to others in whatever way the opportunity presents itself. Look within yourself. Be honest and ask yourself what you need to heal and let go of. Develop a positive perspective and rid yourself of negativity, judgment, and criticism. Practice daily reflection and meditate, exercise, and eat healthy foods. As you adopt healthier ways of living you become a clear intuitive channel and attract positive celestial helpers.

Working with Higher Energies

If the idea of developing medical intuition and accessing higher celestial energies seems a bit overwhelming, take a deep breath and relax. The benevolent healing guides and energies that come to your aid will do all they can to make this as simple for you as possible. In the many years of teaching others to intuitively read the human energy field and invite healing guides to assist them, I have found that it is best to begin by letting go of your expectations. Although most people would like to know their guides' names and utilize them in a particular way, we are usually not in control of this process in the way that we would like.

You will not always know your spirit guides' names and when they are present. Although Dr. Roshi, my health guide, introduced himself to me by name and I recognize when he is with me and helping me, this is more the exception than the rule. I have other spirit guides, angels, and often the spirit guides of my clients that are present when I work. I do not know all of their names and, depending on the health condition and needs of my client, they may come and go of their own accord.

Spirit guides, angels, and even loved ones on the other side will assist you in various ways. Some will amplify your psychic energy, enabling you to better tune in to your health and the health of others. There are guides that will provide more direct assistance and intuitively guide you to problem areas and issues. Others may give you specific medical information. Quite often the client I am working with has a loved one on the other side who is able to provide essential and useful health information and guidance. Other guides and especially angelic helpers will channel healing energy through you to assist in healing.

Many health and healing spirit guides have lived many lives on the earth. They may have been physicians in Eastern and Western medical practices or been part of indigenous and ancient healing traditions. They may have succeeded in mastering various types of healing modalities both in the physical and spiritual realms. They are likely continuing to practice and learn about the healing arts while on the other side. Their help comes to us with no ego involvement or need to be recognized and complimented. Most health and healing guides will be directing, guiding, and helping you without you being aware of their presence.

While you may not always know the name of a helping guide, angel, or loved one on the other side, you can invite loving and wise celestial help and guidance into your medical intuitive work. Simply stating your intent to heal and create good health—mind, body, and spirit—

summons universal healing forces. There is no limit to the kind of help and assistance that you can receive from the spirit realm. Let go and allow the positive flow of wisdom and love to join you.

The spirit guides, loved ones, and angels that help you will choose you based on your needs and your intuitive type. If you are primarily an emotional intuitive you will attract healing helpers who are well versed in accessing and balancing emotional energy. They embody love and are comforting and caring. A mental intuitive attracts wise and understanding spirit guides. They often communicate through thought messages, which may at times be hard to distinguish from your own. Physical intutives often attract earth-based plant and herbal spirits and help from the shamanic realm. They also attract helpers who are able to assist the physical intuitive in moving energy through the body and into conscious awareness. Because of their natural inclination to communicate with the spirit realm, spiritual intuitives may be more aware of their celestial helpers. They are likely to attract guides and angels who are interested and accomplished in the ability to influence and heal the energy field and subtle energies.

Before beginning a medical intuitive session for another or tuning in to your own health, take a moment to ask for the highest love and wisdom from the spirit realm.

Practicing the following meditation will help you to attract and then discern the presence of spirit helpers.

Meditation: Invitation to Spirit Helpers

- Begin by closing your eyes. Slowly inhale and notice your thoughts and emotions. Take note of them and then release them through the outbreath. Continue to breathe in relaxing breath. Move the breath through the body and allow it to relax you. Then exhale any stress or tension through the outbreath.

- Now imagine that you are breathing white light down through the top of the head. Move this breath through the body. Allow it to circulate through your body, loosening and relaxing any stress and tension. Then exhale any stress and tension.

- Take another long white light breath and send this breath into the heart. Breathe cleansing breath into the heart.

- Continue to breathe and relax. Take another long white light breath and imagine that as you exhale you create a white light bubble that completely surrounds you. Continue to breathe and exhale white light energy into this bubble.

- You are safe and protected within this white light bubble. Ask for the presence of a healing guide to enter this white light bubble with you. Continue to breathe, listen, and pay attention to any sensations, feelings, and intuitive thought messages. You may begin to feel a tingling sensation or a sense of alertness and increased energy. You may see flashes of light or an image of the guide or angel who is with you. Pay attention to the slight shifts in energy. Continue to breathe and relax.

- You can send a thought message to this guide. Keep it simple. You can ask their name. But don't let it stall your efforts and receptivity if you do not readily receive one. Not all guides and spirit helpers begin working with you by telling you their names. Some prefer to focus on the work. I have waited for months to know the name of some of my spirit helpers.

- Ask for direction and guidance as you develop medical intuition. Then continue to breathe, relax, and listen. Do not expect too much. Simply be comfortable with the energy and listen and feel.

- When you feel ready, open your eyes and write down all that you experienced. In this way you will ground and strengthen your experience.

Be sure to send gratitude to your health guides and continue to ask for their presence. Even if you do not initially feel that you have made a connection with a guide, give it time. Eventually you will feel their presence and receive useful guidance.

You most likely already have spirit helpers guiding and assisting you. Take your time in getting to know them and pay attention to the surprising and funny ways that they may try to get your attention. Not only are they wise, loving, and helpful, the spirit realm is full of fun and laughter.

In the next chapter you will learn more about other ways that your mind, body, and spirit attempts to get your attention.

16

UTILIZING DREAMS, SYNCHRONICITY, AND ILLNESS AS MESSENGERS

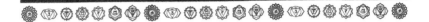

Your mind, body, and spirit are always communicating health information to you. Energy vibrates into conscious awareness. From the unseen, unspoken depths, truth bubbles to the surface. The energy of true health emerges from within and is always intuitively guiding you.

Although we are not always aware of these health messages, your intuition is very resourceful. Energy health information is intuitively communicated in a variety of ways. Some of the most common ways that your mind, body, and spirit communicate to you is through dreams, synchronistic occurrences, and body and health metaphors.

Health Dreams

Intuitive health information may also surface in your dreams. When we sleep the conscious mind is no longer active. This allows our intuitive thoughts and feelings to emerge through our dreams. Important health advice often makes its way into our dream awareness in surprising, often cryptic, and sometimes funny ways. Pay attention to your dreams however nonsensical they may initially appear. They often contain valuable but hidden significance.

It was through a dream that Vera finally found some relief from her migraine headaches. Vera, an office manager in her early fifties, did not know what triggered the shooting and piercing pain that left her debilitated. Several times a month she would retreat to her bedroom, close the curtains, and curl up on her bed. Staying in this position until she felt the pain lift, she did not know what else to do. Not able to tolerate the prescribed medication that her doctor ordered, this seemed to be her only option. One early morning she woke from a deep sleep in the middle of a dream. The dream, she told me, was simple. Vera heard the melody from a popular song repeating itself over and over. But the words of the accompanying verse were different. The next day Vera found herself singing what she heard in the dream: *you make me feel like a magnesium woman.* Although this made her laugh out loud, she knew in her gut that this was more than a hilarious dream. After doing some research on magnesium and migraine headaches she realized the connection. Her headaches, Vera discovered, might be linked to a magnesium deficiency. She headed to a health food store later that day and started taking a magnesium supplement. She felt an immediate improvement. The number and severity of her headaches decreased. Boosted by these positive results, Vera investigated and tried other natural cures. Some helped more than others and the number and intensity of her headaches continued to decrease.

Although Vera was able to recognize that her dream contained a health message, many health-related dreams go unnoticed. At times our dreams point out a health issue in a clear and identifiable way. I once had a dream where an older authoritarian-acting man told me to stop eating chocolate at night if I wanted to sleep better. He was, of course, right. I stopped my nightly dark chocolate treat and my sleep improved. But not all dreams are this clear. Quite often our dreams speak to us in symbolic language and we do not recognize the health message contained within it.

A common symbol in dreams for the physical body is a house. The condition of the walls, floors, and the interior can signify different aspects of your physical self. The foundation of the house is particularly symbolic of the physical body as it represents our core physical stamina and "foundation."

Cars and roads can also symbolize your body and warn of upcoming issues. Pay attention to the condition and the color of the car, as well as the condition of the road and needed repairs. A bumpy uphill road can indicate a difficult time ahead. If you are driving a car that is running out of gas or breaks down, it can be a forewarning of a health issue. I had a dream not long ago of a big car. I was cooking a chicken under the hood. I pulled out a pan of some kind when the chicken was done and placed it back under the hood. The pan continued to sizzle and remain hot, even though I knew the engine was off. When I woke up I realized that the message of the dream was about my health. The car symbolized my moving through life. Cooking was a metaphor for working. The hot pan in the engine told me that I need more down time and rest before I go forward.

Water is often a symbol of our physical, emotional, and spiritual energy. I have had a few dreams of fish tanks and they seem to be good indicators of my energy level. Clear, translucent water is positive energy. A lack of water or cloudy water may be trying to tell you that your physical, emotional, or spiritual energy is low. Hoses, taking a shower or bath, swimming in a dark pool of water or in a tumultuous ocean, and other dream symbols containing water may also have to do with your health. In general, water dreams may indicate the need to physically detox, issues with the lymphatic system, and they can also foretell a pregnancy. Water dreams can also symbolize the need to focus on our emotional and spiritual energy. They may indicate emotional ups and downs and fluctuating energy levels.

Dreams of fire, electrical power lines, digging a hole, mud, an ambulance, medical equipment, hospitals, explosions, lightning, and a hungry baby can be red-flag warnings of a looming health issue. Dreams that foretell healing and physical revitalization often contain positive symbols like flowers blooming, clear skies, calm seas, puppies, rainbows, and pregnancy.

Intuitive Dream Interpretation

Your intuition can be very helpful in interpreting your dreams. Most of the time, we interpret our dreams symbolically. Symbolic dream interpretation explores the meaning behind the predominant dream images. If you suspect that you have had a health-related dream you can further dialogue with the symbols to obtain more information.

Exercise: Symbolic Dream Interpretation

- Write down the dream as soon as you wake up.

- Focus on the predominant symbols.

What symbols provoke the most feeling and reaction within you?

- Close your eyes and imagine one of the symbols.

- Ask it to communicate with you.

Depending on the symbol you can ask such questions as: What are you trying to tell me? What is the feeling associated with this symbol? Is there a health-related message or concern you are trying to make me aware of?

- Use the psychic skills of clairsentience, claircognizance, and clairaudience to receive any other energy information.

- When you have received as much as you can from a symbol, move on to the next predominant one.

- Continue until you have a better understanding of the dream's message.

For example, let's say you had a dream that you were inside a house that you knew was your house, but it looks nothing like your present home or any home you have lived in. After you write down all that you remember about the dream, the color of the house, the condition of it, how you felt within it, close your eyes and speak to the symbols.

For instance, let's say you have a dream that you are living in a house. On the right side of this house the foundation appears to be collapsing.

Close your eyes and take a few deep relaxing breaths.

Imagine an image of the home you saw in your dream and ask it something like, "Why are you crumbling?"

The reply may come through a feeling, a thought, an instantaneous awareness, or you might hear an answer.

Ask more questions of the house if you need further clarification. Continue in the same way with each of the dream images.

Dream Messengers

Loved ones on the other side often share health information with us through our dreams. Friends and family members who have passed over, even those whom we did not know well, are often more aware of our health issues than we are. One of the ways that they try to get our attention and warn and inform us of potential physical issues is at night while we sleep. Sometimes their message is vividly clear and at other times we know the dream's meaning through the emotions and thoughts that it stirs up.

Stanley is a sixty-year-old man who came to the area where I live to lose weight and improve his heath at one of the local health and diet centers. He told me that he had been motivated to focus on improving his health by a visit from his father in a dream. Ill for many years, his father died a few years previous from heart disease.

He told me, "I dreamed that my father was sitting next to my bed. He put his hand to his heart and all of a sudden I was on a lake that we went to when I was young. We had so much fun there. I saw myself as a young man, swimming and water skiing and full of energy. I realized how little energy I now have. I have let myself go for a long time. It felt to me that my father was sending me the message that it was not too late to lose weight and improve my health."

Sometimes the message that a loved one has for us is not easy to decipher. A dream can contain symbolic imagery that does not seem to have much to do with our health. It is important to tune in to your intuition and gut feelings when you are not sure of the dream's meaning. When loved ones and friends on the other side send us information in dreams, it usually comes to us filled with feelings of love and concern. Overall these dreams are more emotional and can leave you feeling as if you had a real encounter with a loved one on the other side.

To better understand a dream that involves a loved one, begin by writing it down. Imagine an image of the loved one that was in the dream. Ask your loved one questions. Their reply may come as an emotional feeling, an instantaneous knowing, or you may hear a message through your inner or outer hearing. If you need further clarification, dialogue with the dream symbols one at a time. A dream dictionary can also provide you with the meaning of common dream symbols. Trust your intuitive gut feeling when interpreting the meaning and message of your dreams.

Exercise: Dream Incubation

You can also invoke and invite dreams that will provide guidance and help in better understanding a health issue or concern. If you would like to receive health and wellness guidance through your dreams, a dreaming technique called dream incubation can be very helpful. Before you go to sleep, contemplate and formulate a conscious intent of what you would like to dream about. You might want to elicit higher guidance on a specific health issue or receive more general wellness guidance. Write down your dream request on a piece of paper and place it under your pillow. Before you go to sleep, intend to remember any dreams that have to do with your request. Have paper and pen near your bed. When you wake, immediately write down any dreams, feelings, and snippets of dreams that you can remember. If you do not have any dreams that night, be patient. Quite often it takes a few days or even weeks to receive and remember the requested guidance through your dreams. Interpret the dreams through the *symbolic interpretation technique* described previously. You might also want to use a dream dictionary to further discern the meaning.

Synchronicity

Synchronicity is an externalized form of intuition. Defined as the coming together of unlikely coincidences, synchronicity is a cosmic exclamation mark informing us of what we need to pay attention to. When you experience a synchronicity, avoid the temptation to dismiss it as meaningless chance or a fluke. This is the universe speaking to you and the warm touch of the divine that tells you that you are being looked after.

I have experienced a few health-related synchronicities that have helped me quite a bit. Several years ago, I had trouble falling and staying asleep. For anyone who suffers from insomnia you know how persistently difficult it can be. One morning after a sleepless night I went to the gym. On the check-in counter was a book about women and hormones. When it came my turn to give the attendant my membership pass, I remarked on the book.

"I just finished it," she told me. "It really helped me with my insomnia. I didn't realize how much hormones can affect our sleep."

"That's interesting," I replied. "I've been struggling with my sleep also. I wonder if my issue is in part hormonal."

"It could be. Why don't you read the book and find out," she suggested. "I see you here all the time. Just return it when you're done."

I took her up on her offer. I started reading the book that evening. It contained suggestions, herbs, and supplements to help with hormones and sleep issues. It helped me tremendously.

Synchronicities can help us in making the best health decisions and choices. It can lead us to the best physicians for our issues, the discovery of uncommon cures for an illness, and assurance that we are on the right track in healing from a health crisis.

Soon after my mother was diagnosed with colon cancer she went through a period of trying to find a doctor with whom she felt comfortable. We went to several different physicians and hospitals. One of the doctors that we went to see worked within a large medical center. We waited for our appointment in a busy waiting area. My mother looked about as lost and miserable as a person in her situation could feel. Slumped in her chair, I knew that she felt hopeless and awkward in this sterile medical setting. As we sat there for what seemed like hours, I suddenly heard my name being called.

"Sherrie, Sherrie, is that you?" I heard from behind the nurses' station. "Honey, what are you doing here?"

In a moment the friendly face of a woman I recognized as having been a client came toward us. I had given Shanice, a woman in her mid-forties, a few readings a year or more previous. I introduced her to my mother and explained that we were there for an appointment with one of the oncologists.

"Oh honey, you come with me," she said to my mother. "I will get you all set up in the back."

Taking my mother's hand, she led her to a small area behind the nurses' station and gave her something to drink. She said to my mother, "Jesus is going to take care of this for you. It's all going to be alright. You'll see. There is a reason for everything. Jesus hasn't forgotten about you. Just give it all over to him."

For some people this kind of assurance might not mean much. But for my mother, a devoutly religious minister, it was exactly what she needed to hear. I watched her stare into the eyes of Shanice. The color in her face came back, her stiff, tight shoulders relaxed, and her vacant eyes softened. I thought that we were in search of the right doctor. Instead, we were led to the right nurse.

Synchronicities come to us in all different ways. The health conversation that you overhear between two women while in an elevator might provide helpful information about a health issue that you have. Spontaneously hearing the name of a particular doctor from several people may be more than a coincidence. Randomly coming across an article while waiting for your car to be fixed that describes new research or treatment for an illness or disease that you or a friend or loved may struggle with may also be an important synchronistic message. In this same way, listen and act when you feel led to reach out, and help and offer support to another who is in a health crisis. You might be their synchronicity.

I had a client who in a couple of days' time had heard of three people who were diagnosed with breast cancer. She thought it more than an odd coincidence and scheduled an appointment for a mammogram. Her test came out fine, but she still had the nagging feeling that there was an important message in this synchronicity. A few nights later she had a dream about her sister. In the dream she saw her sister driving a car with a big dent in the front. Waking from the dream she knew that she needed to call her sister and tell her about the dream and her intuition that something was wrong. Her sister took the dream and her sister's concern seriously and scheduled a mammogram. A small tumor was found in an early stage. After surgery and chemotherapy she is cancer-free.

Illness as a Messenger

There are multidimensional causes and reasons for why we get sick. Most of us are aware that a healthy diet and plenty of exercise contributes in positive ways to our health. We are becoming more aware of the role that our thoughts, attitudes, and emotions have in creating good health and overall well-being. Our connection to our spiritual energy and being in synch with our soul purpose also affects our health. Yet, when we are ill or in pain we tend to primarily focus our attention on the physical causes. We do not always readily consider the emotional, mental, and spiritual influences that may have contributed or be the root cause of our physical issue.

We are energy beings. The physical body is simply a denser vibration of energy. The energy of our thoughts, emotions, and spirit all contribute to our physical health. Before we manifest illness in the physical body, there has already been energetic disharmony. Because we tend to ignore what lies outside of our five senses, the emotional pain, negative attitudes, and spiritual fears that are influencing our health are often easy to dismiss and overlook. This is not true with physical pain. It gets our attention. Our lives are turned upside down when we are physically unable to do the things that we want to do.

When we feel constant discomfort or pain or face a grim prognosis with a life-threatening illness, we are gripped with uncertainty and often fear. We become more willing to pursue whatever will help us to feel better and cure and heal us.

Physical pain and illness can be a messenger. Physical health problems can be a wakeup call, which can inspire and motivate us to grow and evolve spiritually, mentally, and emotionally. Pain and illness alerts us to discover and become conscious of who we are and what we need to pay attention to. It encourages us to expand our awareness of our whole being.

A sacred illness or disease is one in which an illness or disease serves a divine function. This is what is called a soul contract. It is an agreement some souls make before entering the earth life to use illness or disease as a tool for their higher good. When an illness or disease enlightens, transforms, and awakens us to a truth, knowing, and experience of love and compassion that could not come to us any other way, it fulfills a higher purpose.

The idea that the physical body can be a tool that our emotions, mind, and spirit use to awaken us can be hard to accept and fully understand. This is because we believe that we are primarily physical beings. The body defines us and we often believe that without one we cease to exist. Yet, this is simply not true. The body is temporary. The spirit is eternal.

Your spirit will use whatever means necessary to promote your evolution. Sickness and disease can be a vehicle for profound self-awareness. The journey of healing often motivates us to examine our thoughts, emotions, and our spiritual purpose. There are times when the best medical care is not enough. We take the correct medicine and undergo extensive treatments and still we do not heal. Many people who have encountered life-threatening disease and illness and have fully recovered will tell you that healing came about when they focused on non-physical issues.

To heal you might need to release grief, fear, and anger, practice for-giveness, and develop compassion for self and others. It might be nec-essary to dissect your attitudes, negative thoughts, and limited beliefs. Illness can inspire you to embrace your inner power, generate positive energy, and open your heart. Many clients I have worked with radically change their lives as a way to heal. They may develop a new career, leave a marriage or recommit to making one work, pursue an interest that they never had time for, or devote themselves to a spiritual path.

When we are out of synch with our soul purpose and wrapped up in a vicious cycle of creating difficult karma, illness can be a way to get us back on track. Many people who are ill begin to question their life purpose and seek to come into harmony and experience a more peace-ful way of life. I have witnessed many people heal when they approach their illness through this much broader lens. Illness can also lift the veil to the spirit world. Some people discover a connection to the never-ceasing love and comfort of the divine. Their lives transform as they awaken to their true being.

Discerning the Message through the Chakras

One of the reasons that we do not always explore the meaning behind illness is that it can be difficult to decipher. Logic and reasoning does not necessarily provide us with the insight that we need. Your intu-ition, however, can be a powerful ally. It can help you to decipher the symbolic message behind pain, injury, and disease. Discovering what your body is trying to tell you and healing the nonphysical issues will promote full recovery and transformation of the mind, body, and spirit.

The type of illness or physical imbalance that you experience can give important clues as to its associated emotional, mental, and spiri-tual message. There are a few different ways to discern the nonphysi-cal message of an illness or disease. As discussed in previous chapters, the seven chakras each correspond with specific parts of the body, organs, and systems. Each chakra contains the energy imprint of spe-cific emotional, mental, and spiritual lessons and influence. When the flow of vital life force energy through a chakra is blocked or restricted, the physical body suffers and becomes weakened or ill.

The location of physical pain or problems, and the type of illness and disease you have, provides insight into the emotional, mental, and spiritual influences that need to be addressed and healed. Once the underlying issues are known and worked through, the physical body follows suit and heals.

The chart below will guide you to discerning the emotional, mental, and spiritual issues that may be contributing to an illness, pain, or dysfunction. Healing requires rigorous self-examination, honesty, and the willingness to change. If you are experiencing a physical problem, look for the issues associated with it. When you come across an area of concern that you believe may need examination and healing, close your eyes and allow your intuition to guide you. Unlike the conscious self that by nature is often defensive and blind to its own issues and deficits, your spirit can lovingly perceive who we are without shame, guilt, or blame. Ask within if a particular issue is adversely affecting your health, and listen. Emotions, thoughts, spontaneous knowing, and images may surface to further guide you. Continue to listen and intuitively communicate with the energy information that you receive.

Illness, Dysfunction, Imbalance	Associated Emotional, Mental, and Spiritual Issues
First Chakra: Base of the Spine. Varicose veins, prostate problems, rectal and large intestine problems and tumors, base of spine, depression, sciatica, issues with the hips, legs, or feet, frequent illness and immune-related disorders, anorexia, and obesity.	Connection to family and friends and safety and security issues. The ability to ground and live your divine purpose and the power to make positive changes in your life and move forward in your truth.

Illness, Dysfunction, Imbalance (cont.)	Associated Emotional, Mental, and Spiritual Issues (cont.)
Second Chakra: Below Navel. Low back pain, fertility issues, ob/gyn problems, fibroids, uterine cysts, impotence, pelvic pain, libido and urinary problems, intestinal issues, spleen, bladder, appendix, hip problems.	Finances and material success, creativity, passion, and the ability to divinely co-create and manifest our dreams. Guilt, blame, shame, the desire to control others or allowing oneself to be controlled, physical and sexual intimacy, the willingness and ability to act in integrity.
Third Chakra: Solar Plexus. Diabetes, pancreatitis, hepatitis, colon diseases, cirrhosis, digestive imbalances, intestinal tumors, eating disorders, diabetes, hypoglycemia, chronic fatigue, hypertension, muscle spasms and disorders, adrenal fatigue and arthritis. Problems with liver, gallbladder, spleen, middle spine, pancreas.	Issues with personal power, self-esteem, insecurities, stresses, lack of confidence, fears, issues with physical appearance, ambition, sensitivity to criticism, care of self and others, ambition and courage, and our ability to infuse our spiritual essence into our personality.
Fourth Chakra: Chest. Heart disease, breast and lung cancer, lung disease, asthma, fluid in the lungs, issues with the shoulders, arms, and hands, carpal tunnel syndrome, immune disorders, circulatory problems, and issues with the thymus gland.	Emotional fears, vulnerabilities, loneliness, fear, grief, self-centeredness, inability to forgive, and holding on to resentments. Our ability to create balance in the love and care we give to others with the love and care that we give to self. Need to forgive and have gentle compassion for self and others.
Firth Chakra: Throat. Throat cancer, swollen glands, problems with the teeth and gums, laryngitis, chronic sore throat, thyroid issues, joint problems, addictions, issues with the parathyroid, esophagus, hypothalamus.	The ability to speak and express our personal truth, faith, discernment, self-will, the ability to make choices and decisions.

Illness, Dysfunction, Imbalance (cont.)	Associated Emotional, Mental, and Spiritual Issues (cont.)
Sixth Chakra: Between the Brows. Headaches, brain tumors, stroke, neurological disturbances, blindness, deafness, earaches, dyslexia, learning disabilities, seizures, Alzheimer's, mental illness and personality disorders, problems with the pituitary and pineal glands, brain.	Accepting higher truth and wisdom, our ability to open to and accept divine and beneficial spiritual influences, addictive thought patterns, mind chatter, lack of self-evaluation, rejection of new ideas, and feelings of inadequacy and the inability to let go.
Seventh Chakra: Above the Head. Depression, apathy, headaches, sensitivity to light, noise, allergies, multiple sclerosis, epilepsy, Parkinson's disease, senility, schizophrenia, paralysis, dizziness, dissociated states, panic disorders, and nervous and muscular system issues.	Our willingness to surrender to our spiritual purpose and accept and channel our energy into fulfilling our soul plan. Our ability to trust life, be selfless, see the big picture, and contribute to the common good. Over-controlling and over-focus on material gain at the expense of your soul purpose. Stagnation and resistance to change, acceptance or denial of spirituality inspiration and faith.

Uncovering the Message

If you look closely at your aches and pains, illnesses, and physical problem areas, you are likely to discover emotional, mental, and spiritual issues that need your attention. Even the accidents that come our way are often no accident. For instance, the day that my first book came out I took a terrible fall down the stairs outside of my office. Bruised and aching, I was on crutches for weeks with a badly sprained ankle. Even as I stumbled down the stairs, I knew that my fall was no accident. Although I was thrilled to be a published author, I did not know what to expect and I was a bit nervous. The foot lies within the energy of the first chakra. One of the challenges of the first chakra is the ability to move forward. I had been so busy seeing clients and making marketing contacts I had not fully acknowledged my feelings about this step into a more public forum. Now, with this injury, I realized the stress and uncertainty that I had been suppressing. I had to release my belief that I was not a writer and support the shy introvert within me that did not want attention. I knew that I had to listen to my fears and, at the same time, be compassionate and gentle and manage my expectations.

Intuitive

You can also use the *symbolic dream interpretation exercise* as previously described to better discern the energetic cause behind a physical problem or issue. Although an illness does not appear to be symbolic or metaphoric, it often is. If you use the symbolic-interpretation exercise, treat your illness as a dream symbol and communicate with it. Imagine that it has a voice and speak to it. Then listen and pay attention to whatever comes to you. The information that you receive may not be specific to your health. Instead, you might hear a voice that asks you to own your power or make efforts to train for a different job or career. The hardest part of this exercise may be to trust and act on what you receive.

Let go of what you expect to receive. Often the energy behind an illness does not at first make a lot of sense. However, act on what you receive without the need to fully understand it. Ask for suggestions and then follow up and commit to positive action. The results are likely to surprise you with their effectiveness.

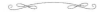

Listening to and understanding the intuitive messages that your mind, body, and spirit sends you can become an enjoyable daily and natural rhythm. Your dreams, synchronicities, and even your aches and pains are speaking to you of a greater experience of wellness and harmony.

In the next chapter deeper avenues of healing through your intuitive type are explored.

17

FURTHER INTUITIVE TYPE
DEVELOPMENT AND HEALING TRAITS

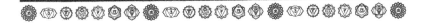

EXERCISE: HEALING TIPS FOR EACH MEDICAL INTUTIVE TYPE

Medical intuition is inherently a form of healing. Medical intuition heals through providing awareness, insight, and knowledge; it also allows for the entry of higher vibration healing energy. Intuition is the voice of your spirit. It connects you to your most powerful self. When you listen to your intuition, wisdom and love flow through you. The healing energy that accompanies a medical intuitive session is silently present, often unacknowledged, yet powerful and pervasive.

Cosmic and divine source healing energy and love flows into the physical realm through those who willingly allow themselves to be used for this purpose. You do not have to be perfect, just willing to allow divine energy to move through you. When we invoke and pray for healing, help, and the presence of higher vibration source energy, this request is met in many ways. There is always an enthusiastic reply and response. Sometimes we directly receive divine intervention and healing. Other times the divine presence and grace comes to us through another. There are angels and benevolent spirits among us who activate the gift of healing and guide us when we are ready to both give and receive healing energy. When you use your intuition to assist others you magnetize to yourself both divine source energy and those who need it and can benefit from it.

A special gift of divine healing energy flows through each intuitive type. Knowing how you can best access your unique healing energy will empower you to better develop its capacity. Remember you are most likely a combination of a few different intuitive types and may identify with more than one of these healing modalities.

EMOTIONAL INTUITIVE HEALING

Emotional intuitives are connected to the divine energy of unconditional love. Engaging, expressive, friendly, and intimate, their open-hearted warmth inspires trust and confidence in others. Emotional intuitives are able to intuitively tune in to emotional wounds, grief, anger, loss, and pain and inject the healing energy of love. Emotional intuitives approach their friends, family, and even strangers with sensitivity and a desire to help and heal. People feel safe and comfortable in their care. Because of their innate intuitive skill of detecting and feeling others' emotional energy, they can uncover the emotional causes behind illness, physical pain, and disease. The confused, suffering, and those in need willingly open their hearts and release their emotional burdens and pain to the emotional intuitive.

Love as Healer

Because of their heartfelt wish to be of service to others, emotional intuitives can sometimes lose their sense of boundaries with their friends, family, and those who they may be helping. They all too often absorb others' emotional pain and difficulties in an attempt to help and heal them. This never works. Absorbing the unresolved emotional energy of others can be overwhelming and cause depression and exhaustion. In addition, when you take on another's emotions, you do not take their pain from them. Instead of unburdening another, the difficult emotions only become stronger. Both you and the person that you wish to help are burdened and locked into experiencing toxic and painful emotions.

One of the biggest lessons an emotional intuitive must learn is to detach from the pain of others. Taking on and absorbing the emotional energy of another is not a solution; sending them forgiveness, unconditional love, and compassion is. If you are an emotional intuitive or have a bit of emotional intuition, know that allowing the higher energy of divine love to flow through you is a more effective form of healing than absorbing others' difficult emotions. Once you experience this kind of transformative healing, it becomes easier to detach and let go of others' pain, grief, and loss. In the beginning of this shift from being an emotional sponge to channeling divine love, you may feel as if you are not doing enough to help others. However, becoming a channel of healing will soon provide you with feelings of freedom and deep healing.

In medical intuitive readings you can intuitively receive energy information and at the same time become a channel of divine love. Set the intent before the session to allow healing energy to flow through you. In this way, as you scan yourself or do other intuitive exercises, you also heal. If you are giving a medical intuitive reading to another and you feel yourself being drawn into their emotional energy, resist the temptation to take on their burdens. Remind yourself that you can better help your client by maintaining a higher level of consciousness. Stay focused in the energy of love, allowing higher positive vibrations to naturally flow through you.

Emotional Clearing

Emotional intuitives can also get lost and overwhelmed in their own emotions and complex emotional nature. It can be helpful to balance the tendency to focus on emotional energy by engaging in mental, physical, and spiritual intuitive energy preferences. For instance, use the mental intuitive's natural claircognizant knowing to understand the emotional influences affecting you, or the physical intuitive's gift of connectedness to nature to illicit inner calm and serenity.

If you are an emotional intuitive, you have an innate connection to the angelic realm. Daily conscious connection through meditation and invoking the presence of angels can also be beneficial in maintaining a higher frequency of love energy. Many of the emotional intuitives that I know are surrounded with angels who on a daily basis channel healing love to them and through them to those in need. Angels do not absorb our negativity, pain, and stress. Instead they lift us into higher realms of comfort, inspiration, peace, and well-being. This higher source energy vibration can transform your pain into joy and your negativity into positivity.

Accept the angelic unconditional love and healing energy that is being broadcast your way. Take time every day to contemplate the beauty and power of love and know that you are in the company of angels. Open your heart and discharge the difficult emotions and fill yourself with divine love. Love is your greatest teacher. It will guide, heal, and restore your mind, body, and spirit.

MENTAL INTUITIVE HEALING

Mental intuitives find their inspiration and joy in the realm of pure consciousness. No idea and possibility is lightly dismissed and too far-fetched for the mental intuitive to consider. With a broad view of reality, they accumulate and accept all truths. Driven to know and understand, their intuition is relentlessly probing. The mental intuitive's gift of heal-ing springs from their comprehensive and far-reaching intuitive per-ception. With the ability to intuit the interconnectedness between the body, mind, and spirit, they heal through awareness, knowledge, and wisdom.

Steps to Mastery

Mental intuitives by nature tend to be objective and reserved. They do not jump into others' emotions the way emotional intuitives do. They are more likely to dissect and understand than feel and emote. If you are a mental intuitive it is important to treat yourself with compas-sion, love, and forgiveness. You may tend to be self-critical and your expectations for yourself can, at times, be too high and demanding. Pay attention to your emotions and allow yourself to become aware of and express difficult and repressed feelings such as grief, fear, and sadness, even when you do not feel as if it is rational or logical. This will invite and generate mind, body, and spirit healing and revitalization.

People may often feel known, seen, and acknowledged in your presence. Your desire to intuit, see, and know all can either bring reassurance to others or leave them feeling exposed and vulnerable. As you use your gifts to better understand yourself, you will be able to direct this loving, wise awareness to others. As a medical intuitive your challenge is to cultivate personal sensitivity and responsiveness to your clients. Emotional intuitives can absorb and get lost in others' emotions. A mental intuitive can get equally lost in intuited information and over-thinking. Others may not be able to follow your reasoning, logic, and comprehensive explanations. Decoding and sharing what you have intuitively received is not always easy. Address your client personally and with compassion. Keep your explanations specific, concise, and understandable. If your client has questions, you can go into more detailed and extensive explanations.

The Healing Mind

Mental intuitives operate from the belief that the mind is the healer. When intuitively alert they are able to intuit the beliefs, thoughts, and attitudes that negatively impact health. Because they inherently understand how thoughts influence health, they can use this penetrating awareness and power to transform their negativity and limited beliefs and inspire others to do the same.

Mental intuitives often practice and motivate others to use positive thinking and affirmations as a transformative tool. Affirmations are short, powerful statements. When you say or think one repeatedly, the statement becomes the thought that creates your reality. Affirmations can become the energy through which your mind, body, and spirit attracts and generates positive health and well-being. Mental intuitives have an innate connection to divine mind and tend to be strong-willed and focused. Because mind and thought is their conduit for divine energy, they can benefit from affirmations in a more direct and effective way than the other types.

You can use affirmations in every area of your life. When it comes to your health, an effective general overall healing affirmation may be something as simple as:

I am full of energy and vitality, my body is strong and healthy.

Or you can focus on one area of health and well-being, such as:

My heart radiates with love and perfect health.

Affirmations are most effective when they are spoken aloud or written down repetitively over the course of an extended period of time.

Along with affirmations, other mindful practices such as hypnosis and meditation are often utilized by mental intuitives for mind, body, and spirit healing. More than the other types of intuitives, mental intuitives are attracted to innovative healing techniques and systems that offer new technology. Quite often they are the ones developing and inventing unique methods and tools for healing. As medical intuitives, mental intuitives often develop penetrating X-Ray intuitive sight. They are able to perceive the interplay of the different systems of the body almost as if they are reading a blueprint.

A mental intuitive is at their best when they rely on their intuition and do not overthink the energy information they receive. This may always be somewhat of a temptation. Accepting what you intuit without being able to fully understand it can be a challenge. When working with others, finding the balance between simply stating what is intuitively perceived without overanalyzing it will produce the best and most accurate intuitive reading. Enlightening ah-ha moments of penetrating insights can bring about instantaneous transformation. Once you experience this, you will likely better trust your pure intuitive insights.

Higher Consciousness

As channels of higher consciousness, mental intuitives often receive energy information from higher forms of intelligence. These more evolved life forms are often nonphysical beings that willingly assist the human world in evolution and healing. Mental and spiritual intuitives are attracted to conversing and communicating with other planetary life, and it is the mental intuitive that has the easiest time deciphering and understanding these communications.

Mental intuitives are also likely to know a bit about the source of their intuitive information. Unlike the other types of intuitives, mental intuitives want to know where the healing energy is coming from, why it is, and how to best utilize it. The same is true for their ability to channel source healing energy. With their tendency to overanalyze, it can be challenging to accept, feel, and allow pure divine healing energy to flow through them to others. For this reason, it can be beneficial for a mental intuitive to regularly meditate and intuitively connect with higher source healing energy in order to become more familiar and comfortable with it.

If you are a mental intuitive, pure awareness will reveal all truth for you. In truth lies your freedom, connection to source energy, and enlightened healing. Take time every day to seek beyond illusion and conventionality and into the root and mystery of all that is. This is where you will discover your deepest self and ultimate healing.

Physical Intuitive Healing

Physical intuitives are at home in the body. Just as emotional intuitives innately tune in to emotions and mental intuitives tune in to thoughts, physical intuitives have a natural intuitive and spiritual connection with the physical world. Unlike the other types, their intuition emerges through their five senses. Their sight, hearing, and touch penetrate beyond physical boundaries and into energy awareness and insight. For instance, a physical intuitive might notice a slight imbalance in the way that someone walks. From this observation he or she might be intuitively led to a weakness in the hip that feels stiff or brittle. It might not seem to the physical intuitive that this is intuitive information. Instead, they would argue it is just simple observation and logic.

Physical intuitives are natural hands-on healers. Their hands both receive intuitive energy information and transmit cosmic healing. Although they are intuitively attuned to the finer vibrations of energy inherent in all physical matter, they may have a difficult time adequately communicating what their hands so easily intuit. For this reason, physical intuitives are attracted to less communicative healing modalities such as massage, healing touch, and Reiki. Their hands know where to go and what to do.

Becoming Aware

The challenge for a physical intuitive is to become conscious of and put words to the energy information that they receive. They tend to be practical, unassuming, and down-to-earth. Not given over to displays of wit and wisdom, they like to get the job done, simply and easily. Explaining what they have intuitively received may be a challenge that they are not always comfortable with. However, when they do venture into the world of words, their explanations tend to be concise and direct. Unlike the mental intuitive that may overanalyze and overthink intuitive information, physical intuitives simply report what they have seen, felt, heard, or experienced with as few words as possible. Another charming aspect of physical intuitives is that they do not mind being "wrong" in their intuitive perceptions. Mental intuitives can take an intuitive misstep too seriously and begin to doubt their competency. A physical intuitive may only shrug their shoulders and not be too surprised that their words failed them. They likely will surmise that they have intuited the correct information but explained it ineffectively.

Intuiting Through the Hands

If you are a physical intuitive or score high on physical intuition, you may want to include a hand scan as part of a medical intuitive body scan. Along with intuitively dialoguing with your energy through clairvoyance and the other psychic skills, use your physical sensitivity to intuit. Place your hands on the part of your body that you are scanning. As an intuitive sensor your hands will feel and receive the energy information that is being emitted. When you use your hands to intuit in this way, they can also be a conduit for healing energy.

If you use a hand scan when working with others it is important to not transmit your personal energy to them. It is exhausting to heal in this way and you run the risk of receiving others' energy. To activate divine source healing energy during a hands-on scan for yourself or others, simply state that this is your intent and take a moment to feel a warm or tingly flow of energy move through you before beginning the session.

Physical intuitives connect with the divine energy within all living things. When ill, feeling low energy, or to maintain good health, herbs, plants, crystals, and animal spirit medicine offer a divine and healing tincture. Communing with nature, having pets or animals nearby, or walking next to the seashore or under the stars regularly also maintains health and well-being. Being in nature can also be a useful way to discharge accumulated negative and absorbed energy within the body. Because of the physical intuitive's tendency to unknowingly take on the energy of others and their aches and pains, they need to remember to clear their body of any nonbeneficial energy that they may have unknowingly absorbed.

If you are a physical intuitive and ill or feeling a lack of energy, try this:

Hold a crystal, sit next to a river, against a tree trunk, or close to any natural source of energy. Close your eyes, and through vibrational sensitivity, feel the flow of vital life force energy. Open yourself and receive the healing energy and natural divine spirit of the elements. Imagine toxins and energy that you no longer need dissipating and evaporating as revitalizing life force energy moves through you.

More than the other types of intuitives, you live in the world of matter and spirit as one force. Enjoy and indulge yourself in this innate wisdom. Experience the cosmic love and healing energy as it flows through the breeze, shines down on you from the stars, and peeks at you through the eyes of a deer. This is your healing.

Spiritual Intuitive Healing

Spiritual intuitives are less concerned than the other intuitive types with the purely physical realm. They are, however, interested in and intuitively attuned to energy. Unlike the physical intuitive, a spiritual intuitive does not have a natural affinity for the material realm and the physical body. They, of course, understand its usefulness and importance, but they do not necessarily have a desire to work within what appears to be its solid and concrete parameters. However, once spiritual intuitives perceive the body as energy, this bias often changes. Those spiritual intuitives that pursue developing medical intuition are often motivated to do so by their ability to perceive the physical body as a flowing network of colorful and intricate energy.

Attuning to the Higher Realms

A spiritual intuitive has a tangible connection to the spirit realms. Of all of the intuitive types, spiritual intuitives are more likely to enjoy communicating, visiting, and conversing with nonphysical beings. They do this through what may appear to the other types to be whimsical and fanciful meanderings.

If you are a spiritual intuitive pay attention to your daydreams and playful imagination as there is often more power in these states than you may realize. Your interest in otherworldly pursuits and the supernatural, mystical, and spiritual realms may be a calling to higher awareness and conscious connection with spiritual realms. As you continue to develop your intuitive gifts and your natural connection to higher states of energy, you will activate your natural ability to perceive auras and consciously converse and learn from and visit with spirit helpers. More at home with pure essence and energy than the other intuitive types, your intuitive sensors tend to be able to differentiate and identify the varied forms of nonphysical life. Because of this, your ability to work with higher vibrational healing forces is more developed than the other types.

Connection to Spirit Guides and the Other Side

Of all of the intuitive types, spiritual intuitives are most likely to desire to become aware of and know who their spirit guides are and who on the other side may be helping them. They often receive healing guidance and assistance through their dreams, meditation, and instantaneous awareness. Even when they do not know their spirit helpers' names, or they cannot readily identify the spirit presence that they intuit close by, there is a familiar and comforting intuitive sense that they are not alone and that they can trust their elusive visitors.

As medical intuitives, spiritual intuitives often wholeheartedly invite the presence of spirit helpers to assist them in understanding their health and intuiting energy information. Whether it is angels, spirit guides, divine presence, or a loved one on the other side, they are comfortable with cosmic help and healing. A spiritual intuitive may have a specific spirit guide who works with them on a continual basis or a few that come and go based on the current needs. Because of their ease with working with guides, angels, and pure source energy, many spiritual intuitives further develop and become gifted energy healers.

When it comes to health energy information, spiritual intitives are likely to intuitively perceive less physically tangible energy information than the other intuitives. Psychic disturbances such as past lives, negative attachments, and issues with the chakras and energy field are likely to get the spiritual intuitive's psychic attention. Unlike physical intuitives, who skillfully hone in on the more physical aspects of the body, like the organs and the various systems, spiritual intuitives are experts at detecting energetic issues. Because they are primarily focused in higher nonphysical vibrations, spiritual intutives may need to remind themselves to focus on the more dense aspects of the physical body.

The Here and Now

The challenge for many spiritual intuitives lies in their ability to live in the physical here and now and discover their purpose on earth. Because they enjoy altered states of awareness and the lofty realms of pure energy, they may have a harder time finding meaningful work and an avenue for their natural gifts. It can be helpful for the spiritual intuitive to practice and take on some of the physical intuitives' innate characteristics. Spending time in nature, feeling the divine with all forms of life, can help them to better appreciate and find meaning in this world.

If you are a spiritual intuitive, it can be helpful to realize that all of physical life at its most authentic root is spiritual energy. Look within yourself to understand what your unique contribution to others and to this earth may be and pursue it with the same interest and drive that you use to pursue connection with the higher energy realms.

Spiritual intuitives heal through invoking and generating positive and divine vibrations of energy. Of all of the intuitive types they are the most comfortable with working with pure energy. If you are a spiritual intuitive, you may need to regularly focus on circulating divine source energy throughout the physical body. In this way you become a powerful force and pillar of strength and awareness for yourself and others by uniting the divine and physical realms.

MEDITATION: EARTH AND SKY ENERGY HEALING

With a tender ease and sublime enjoyment, your ability to mingle with cosmic and divine energy can benefit you, others, and the planet. First you must channel it into the body. This exercise can help you to transfer your cosmic lofty vibrations to the here and now. This meditation is also useful for all of the intuitive types to regularly absorb healing energy and integrate it throughout the body, mind, and spirit.

You can practice this mediation throughout the day, when you are feeling low energy, or are ill or in pain or just want to revitalize yourself.

Close your eyes, stand with your feet about shoulder-width apart, and your arms at your side.

Visualize a rainbow of colored energy moving up from the earth and down through the top of your head. Breathe in this energy and move it through your body in a figure-eight pattern, down one side of the body and at your solar plexus moving up the other side. You may feel a slight tingling or buzzing feeling throughout your body as the energy moves through you.

Open the palms of your hands and turn them upward. Through clairvoyant perception, see the energy move into the palms of your hands—visualize a rainbow of energy move through the palms of your hands. Imagine your hands filling with this energy. You may feel a tingling, or even a sensation of heat, as the energy flows to and collects in your hands.

Move one of your hands above your head, palm facing the top of your head. Feel white light energy being transmitted through your palm into your body.

Place your other hand over your third eye and visualize purple energy streaming through your palm and into your third eye. Hold this position for a moment and breathe long, deep breaths.

Now place both of your hands over your heart, with your palms facing the heart. Visualize green energy streaming from your palms and into your heart. Feel this energy move through you. Breathe in this healing green energy.

When you are ready place both of your palms on your solar plexus, and visualize green, white, and purple energy moving through your palms and into your solar plexus. Feel the power of this energy move through you. Breathe in this healing energy and feel it circulate through your body.

When you are ready place your hands to your side with your palms open toward the earth. Visualize red, orange, and yellow energy moving up through your palms. Breathe and increase the vibration of the energy moving through your palms.

Place your palms on your solar plexus and feel the red, yellow, and orange energy move through your body. Continue to breathe in this energy through your palms. Feel this circulate through your body.

When you are ready, move your arms to your side with one palm facing toward the earth and the other facing toward the sky, visualize a rainbow of healing color energy move through your body. Feel yourself as energy, grounded to the earth and a channel for cosmic high vibration. Breathe and send your healing energy to anyone who may need it and send it to the planet.

You can practice calling in this healing anywhere, at various times throughout the day. This meditation will lovingly connect your spirit to the earth, fortify your physical body, and refresh your spirit.

Accessing higher states of awareness, wisdom, and love where illness, pain, and disease cease to exist, and channeling this vibration into the world of physicality is the special gift of the spiritual intuitive. Sail into these sublime states and don't forget to share it with us.

Developing the healing potential inherent with your intuitive type is a personal decision. There are many avenues and potent sources of love and wisdom that are present to support and guide you along the way. At times healing gifts emerge naturally and at other times it is a more conscious choice to explore and learn new techniques. Either way, trust yourself and listen to your intuition and allow it to open new doors of health and well-being.

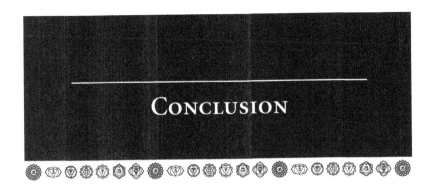

CONCLUSION

Medical Intuition: Its Never-Ending Gift

At the beginning of the journey of developing medical intuition, you may feel as if your intuition is somewhat like a little spring seed sprout. Gently shooting up from the dark earth and peeking into the light of day, the invisible force of growth transforming the seed into the daisy or the oak tree. So it is with your natural intuitive ability. Like a seed, your intuitive ability has immense potential. There is a silent force within you that knows who you are and what you are capable of. I hope that while reading this book you have caught a glimpse of it. Developing your medical intuition is more than simply learning an interesting skill. It is a journey that can inspire you to fully awaken to the power that resides and has always resided within you. Your intuition is the voice of this power as it speaks to you from the deep recess of your spirit. You have more power to heal your mind, body, and spirit than you have been led to believe. As you activate this knowing, new insights and miraculous healing will become the norm.

Your Changing Medical Intuitive Type

You may have begun this journey by discovering that you are an emotional, mental, physical, or spiritual intuitive. However your intuition initially surfaces, as you develop medical intuition you will utilize and further develop all of the four types. As you do this, you not only increase your intuitive ability, you also expand your awareness as to how others experience their intuition. Tapping into the various ways that intuition surfaces empowers you to use your intuition on a daily basis for your everyday concerns and for spiritual development.

My books *Discover Your Psychic Type, Love and Intuition,* and *You are a Medium,* all utilize the framework of intuitive types. One of the most common questions I am asked by readers of these books is if intuitive types can change over time and if it is common to have more than one predominant type. Your intuitive type is fluid and adaptable. Not only do you intuit through more than one type, your type will change according to your intuitive focus. For instance, my predominant intuitive type in the area of love and relationships is spiritual and emotional. My predominant type in medical intuition is mental and spiritual. The optimum is to be able to consciously use all four types.

You Are Supported

There is a silent conspiracy at work with intuitive awareness. We use it for the practical concerns of our material day-to-day life. Yet, like the silent seed, it has its own design and purpose. As you develop and expand your intuition, your spirit unfolds, branches out, and connects with the physical and spiritual realms in a new and more all-embracing way. Like the flower and the small oak, your leaves and branches feel the light of the sun and the warm breeze lifting you out of the darkness.

There is an undeniable paradox that you may experience while developing and practicing medical intuition. While medical intuition is focused in the physical body, it offers a surprising connection with the cosmic forces. There is an invisible source of healing that supports your efforts. Maybe you have experienced this for yourself. The cosmos know only health. It is only here on earth that we experience illness, pain, and decline. When we begin to communicate with energy and use our intuition for the purpose of healing we tap into a powerful reality. Your efforts to elicit the strength, wisdom, and love within your spirit connects you to a community of divine help.

Modern medicine, for the most part, treats the physical body as if it is separate and more powerful than the invisible force within it. Medical intuition reverses this concept. It wakes us to the awareness that the body is simply the manifestation of a much more potent energy force. As this truth unfolds, you eventually come to realize a personal truth. No longer will you be able to perceive yourself as a powerless pawn in the game of life. You discover the spirit within and confront the knowledge that you are connected to a much more vast, intelligent, and loving source than anything that you may have encountered in the physical world. Once you become aware of this inner power you are taken to the doorway of transformation. You have a choice. You can either believe in the power within or the power of the external world. It is at this point that your intuition weakens and hesitates, or strengthens and reveals deeper sources of wisdom and love.

Allow the Light to Shine Through You

To be an effective medical intuitive you have to accept your inner power. The accuracy and reliability of your intuitive ability is directly connected to your willingness to embrace a greater you. Most people unknowingly limit their intuitive abilities.

Children are naturally intuitive. Most people have had some form of intuitive encounter or experience of extrasensory perception as a child. Yet, few parents and schools acknowledge and create a safe opportunity for young people to share and express these experiences. Feeling isolated and alone and unable to understand what they are experiencing, many children suppress their intuition out of fear that they are different or that there is something wrong with them.

To fully reactivate your intuition you must let go of your fear and become comfortable with your personal power. This power is not your ego. It is the greater part of you. It is your spirit, the eternal source of wisdom and love within. Get out of the way and allow a stronger ray of light to shine through. So many times in readings a part of me wants to resist letting go and deferring to a higher source.

Yet, I know that the energy information that I receive will be much more useful and accurate if I just quietly listen and receive. I have to quiet the ego part of me that wants to take charge. The ego will always want center stage and will try and convince you that you do not have the innate ability to intuit your or another's health. You do.

Live in Balance and Joy

Accepting your natural intuition, developing it, and using it to help yourself and others will change you. You may have initially been motivated to develop medical intuition to better tune in to your health or the health of others. You may work in a field where you already care for others and you would like to use your intuition in a beneficial way. You might be a massage therapist, an acupuncturist, a chiropractor, or work in one of the many similar fields. You may be a professional intuitive, healer, tarot card reader, or spiritual or metaphysical teacher. Perhaps your job or career does not appear to be very "spiritual." It may not give you an opportunity to directly help others. Maybe you work in an office, at home, in a health care facility, a school, or a factory. It doesn't matter where you work or what you do. Whatever has attracted you to develop medical intuition or whatever you presently do for a career, activating your ability to intuitively tune in to your health and heal yourself and others will open unseen doors and opportunities.

You now emit a wise and loving light that magnetizes those in need. An invisible current attracts those who you can help, either in a professional or nonprofessional way. Even if you read this book to intuitively tune in to your own health, without the thought of helping others, your friends, family, and others will seek you out. It is essential that you accept this divine gift of service, but first and foremost, commit to caring for yourself. Resist becoming overwhelmed with others' expectations and demands. Love yourself, treat yourself with gentle compassion, and maintain your serenity and peace of mind. You cannot help others if you are not living a life of balance and joy.

There are many who may need your help. But there are many who can also provide the help that others may need. The power that moves through you moves through everyone. Some are more aware of it than others. Yet, even when we do not know that we have the power within to heal and live in joy and peace, it is still there. When you know this about others and reflect it back to them you help them to perceive it in themselves. Appreciate your contributions and the contributions of others. Be kind, compassionate, and loving, and the world and the realm of all love, peace, and joy will show up at your door and give you the same.

Appendix 1

SCANNING PROCESS AND LOCATION OF ORGANS

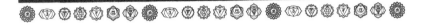

- Starting at the seventh chakra above the head, scan the energy field or aura.

- Continue to the sixth chakra and scan the brain, the sinus and face, the eyes and nose, then the ears and teeth.

- Then scan the fifth chakra: the neck, the throat, the shoulders, and then the arms and hands.

- Proceed to the fourth chakra: the heart, the bronchial tubes, the lungs, and the breasts.

- Then scan the third chakra: the stomach, the gallbladder on the right side (left side when scanning another), the liver on the right side (left side for another), the spleen on the left side (right side for another), and then the pancreas on the left side (right side for another).

- Scan the second chakra: the colon, which lies across stomach; if you are a woman, scan the ovaries on the right and left side, and the uterus; and if you are a man the testes and prostate; and then the bladder low center.

- Proceed to the first chakra: scan the spine, the right and left kidney, lower colon, and the legs and the feet.

- Then scan the endocrine system: the adrenals, then the thymus, thyroid, pituitary, and the pineal.

- Scan the lymphatic system, the circulatory system, the nervous system, and the skeletal system.

Bibliography & Reading List

Chapter 1

Jouanna, Jacques. *Hippocrates.* Baltimore, MD: Johns Hopkins University Press, 1999.

Sugrue, Thomas. *There Is a River,* revised edition. Virginia Beach, VA: A.R.E. Press, January 1, 1997.

Chapter 2

Andrews, Ted. *How to Heal with Color.* Minneapolis, MN: Llewellyn Publications, November 8, 2005.

Dale, Cyndi. *The Subtle Body: An Encyclopedia of Your Energetic Anatomy.* Louisville, CO: Sounds True, February 2009.

Eden, Donna, David Feinstein, Brooks Garten. *Energy Medicine.* New York, NY: Jeremy P. Tarcher/Putnam, December 27, 1999.

Chapter 4

Ody, Penelope. *The Chinese Medicine Bible: The Definitive Guide to Holistic Healing.* New York, NY: Sterling Publishing, 2011.

Shealy, Norman. *Medical Intuition: Your Awakening to Wholeness.* Virginia Beach, VA: 4th Dimension Press, August 18, 2010.

Chapter 5

Sugrue, Thomas. *There Is a River*, revised edition. Virginia Beach, VA: A.R.E. Press, January 1, 1997.

Merriam-Webster. *Merriam-Webster's Collegiate Dictionary*, 10th Edition. New York, NY: Merriam-Webster, 1998.

Holmes, Ernest. *The Science of Mind: Complete and Unabridged.* Radford, VA: Wilder Publications, February 19, 2010.

Hay, Louise. *You Can Heal Your Life.* Santa Monica, CA: Hay House, 1984.

Chapter 7

Eden, Donna, David Feinstein, and Brooks Garten. *Energy Medicine.* New York, NY: Jeremy P. Tarcher/Putnam, December 27, 1999.

Chapter 8

Myss, Caroline. *Anatomy of the Spirit: The Seven Stages of Power and Healing.* New York, NY: Harmony, August 26, 1997.

Dale, Cyndi. *The Subtle Body: An Encyclopedia of Your Energetic Anatomy.* Louisville, CO: Sounds True, February 2009.

Chapter 10

Dale, Cyndi. *The Subtle Body: An Encyclopedia of Your Energetic Anatomy.* Louisville, CO: Sounds True, February 2009.

Eden, Donna, David Feinstein, and Brooks Garten. *Energy Medicine.* New York, NY: Jeremy P. Tarcher/Putnam, December 27, 1999.

Ody, Penelope. *The Chinese Medicine Bible: The Definitive Guide to Holistic Healing.* New York, NY: Sterling Publisher, August 2012.

Chapter 11

Judith, Anodea. *Wheels of Life: A User's Guide to the Chakra System.* Minneapolis, MN: Llewellyn Publications, 1987.

Myss, Caroline. *Anatomy of the Spirit: The Seven Stages of Power and Healing.* New York, NY: Harmony, August 26, 1997.

Dale, Cyndi. *The Subtle Body: An Encyclopedia of Your Energetic Anatomy.* Louisville, CO: Sounds True, February 2009.

Eden, Donna, David Feinstein, Brooks Garten. *Energy Medicine.* New York, NY: Jeremy P. Tarcher/Putnam, December 27, 1999.

Chapter 12

Brennan, Barbara. *Hands of Light: A Guide to Healing Through the Energy Field.* New York, NY: Bantam, May 1, 1988.

Myss, Caroline. *Anatomy of the Spirit: The Seven Stages of Power and Healing.* New York, NY: Harmony, August 26, 1997.

Dale, Cyndi. *The Subtle Body: An Encyclopedia of Your Energetic Anatomy.* Louisville, CO: Sounds True, February 2009.

Chapter 16

Myss, Caroline. *Anatomy of the Spirit: The Seven Stages of Power and Healing.* New York, NY: Harmony, August 26, 1997.

Dale, Cyndi. *The Subtle Body: An Encyclopedia of Your Energetic Anatomy.* Louisville, CO: Sounds True, February 2009.

Chapter 17

Andrews, Ted. *How to Heal with Color.* Minneapolis, MN: Llewellyn Publications, November 8, 2005.

Myss, Caroline. *Anatomy of the Spirit: The Seven Stages of Power and Healing.* New York, NY: Harmony, August 26, 1997.

Reading List

Let Magic Happen: Adventures in Healing with a Holistic Radiologist. Larry Burke. Durham, NC: Healing Imager Press, June 2102.

Dream Dictionary. Tony Crisp. New York, NY: Dell, January 29, 2002.

You Can Heal Your Life. Louise Hay. Santa Monica, CA: Hay House, 1984.

Energy Medicine. Donna Eden, David Feinstein, and Brooks Garten. New York, NY: Jeremy P. Tarcher/Putnam, December 27, 1999.

The Subtle Body: An Encyclopedia of Your Energetic Anatomy. Cyndi Dale. Louisville, Colorado: Sounds True, February 2009.

Anatomy of the Spirit: The Seven Stages of Power and Healing. Caroline Myss. New York, NY: Harmony, August 26, 1997.

How to Heal with Color. Ted Andrews. Minneapolis, MN: Llewellyn Publications, November 8, 2005.

Hands of Light: A Guide to Healing Through the Energy Field. Barbara Brennan. New York, NY: Bantam, May 1, 1988.

Wheels of Life: A User's Guide to the Chakra System. Judith Anodea. Woodbury, MN: Llewellyn Publications, 1987.

Discover Your Psychic Type: Developing and Using Your Natural Intuition. Sherrie Dillard. Woodbury, MN: Llewellyn Publications, 2008.

The Miracle Workers Handbook: Seven Levels of Power and Manifestation of the Virgin Mary. Sherrie Dillard. United Kingdom: John Hunt Publishing, 2012.

How to See and Read the Aura. Ted Andrews. Woodbury, MN: Llewellyn Publications, 2006.

Chinese Healing Exercises: A Personalized Practice for Health & Longevity. Steven Cardoza. Woodbury, MN: Llewellyn Publications, November 2013.

The Healing Power of Reiki: A Modern Master's Approach to Emotional, Spiritual & Physical Wellness. Raven Keyes. Woodbury, MN: Llewellyn Publications, October 2012.

The Chinese Medicine Bible: The Definitive Guide to Holistic Healing. Penelope Ody. New York, NY: Sterling Publisher, August 2012.

Acknowledgments

In gratitude to Dr. Barbara Burggraaff, Dr. Larry Burke, for his passion for medical intuition, and Dr. Roshi, who has taught me so much. Thank you to those who, over the years, trusted my intuitive insight into their health and wellbeaing.

Many thanks to Angela Wix, for her insight and confidence; not all acquisitions editors are equal and she is the best. Thank you to Patti Frazee, for her clarity and fantastic editing skills, Kat Sanborn, and the hard working folks at Llewellyn.

To Write to the Author

It has been a joy to share my psychic and medium adventures with you. You inspire, motivate, and teach me. I would love for you to share your insights and experiences with me.

You can e-mail me at sgd7777@yahoo.com or go to my website, www.sherriedillard.com, and sign up for my newsletter for updates. I also invite you to follow me on Facebook, www.facebook.com /sherrie.dillard.

—Sherrie Dillard